Mike Samuels, M.D., and Nancy Samuels

The well child coloring book

A child's guided tour through the body
How it works, how to keep it healthy

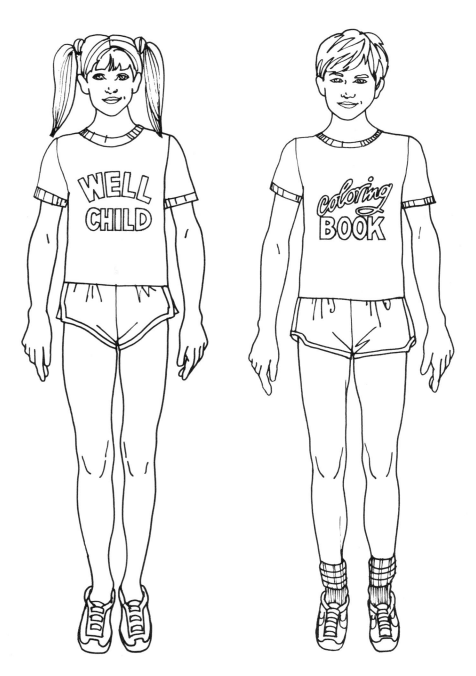

Drawings by Wendy Frost

Summit Books   New York

Published by SUMMIT BOOKS

A Simon & Schuster Division
of Gulf & Western Corporation

Simon & Schuster Building
Rockefeller Center
1230 Avenue of the Americas
New York, New York 10020

SUMMIT BOOKS and colophon
are trademarks of Simon & Schuster

Designed by Clint Anglin

Manufactured in the
United States of America

10 9 8 7 6 5 4 3 2 1

First Edition

ISBN 0–671–45466–8

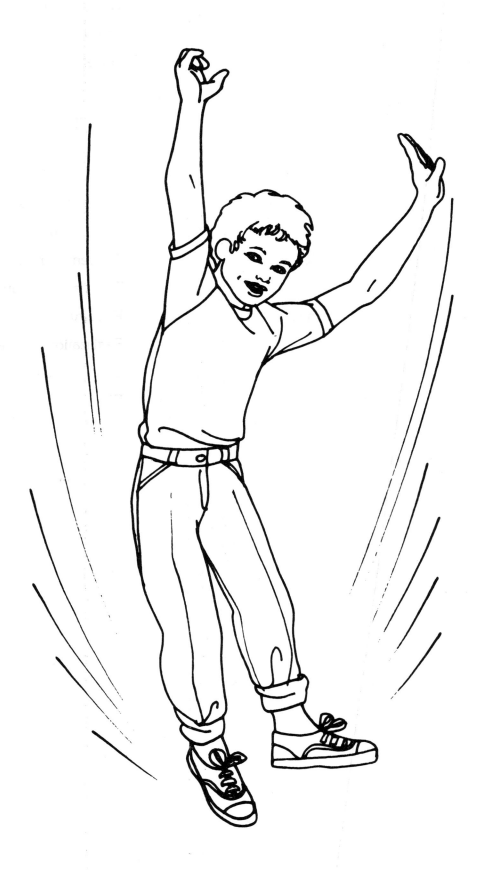

Contents

The cell   2

Cell division   3

The skeleton   4

How bones grow   6

The joints   7

The tooth   8

Tooth eruption   9

The muscles   10

How muscles move   12

Temperature regulation   13

The skin   14

Skin messages and the fingernails   15

The digestive system   16

The villi and the liver   17

The respiratory system   18

The vocal cords and the cilia   19

Breathing in and out   20

How air gets into the blood   21

The circulatory system   22

Arteries and veins   23

The capillaries and blood composition   24

How the heart pumps   25

The lymph system   26

How a lymph node works   27

The urinary system   28

How the kidney works   29

The nervous system   30

The brain and the spinal cord   31

Reflexes   32

The nerve cell and the synapse   33

The autonomic nervous system   34

The eye   35

The eye muscles and tears   36

How the eye focuses   37

The ear   38

The nose   40

The tongue   41

The endocrine system   42

How thoughts affect the endocrine system   43

The female reproductive system   44

The male reproductive system   45

Puberty   46

Fertilization of an egg   48

Growth of a baby   49

Blood clotting   50

Skin healing   51

Bone healing   52

How antibodies destroy bacteria   53

How stress affects the body   54

How relaxation affects the body   55

How to relax   56

How to use mind pictures   57

Healthy eating   58

Unhealthy eating   59

Body pollution   60

How aerobic exercise affects the body   61

Feeling good   62

The cell

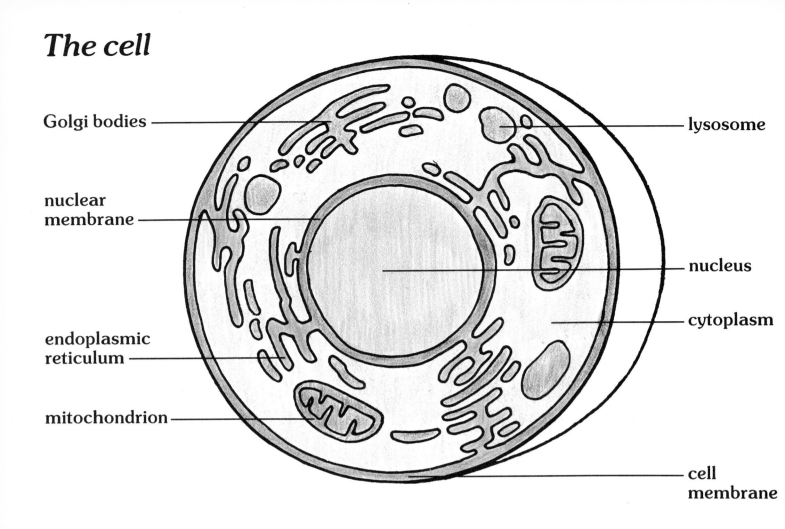

Golgi bodies

nuclear membrane

endoplasmic reticulum

mitochondrion

lysosome

nucleus

cytoplasm

cell membrane

The cell Cells are the building blocks of the body. They come in different shapes and sizes and they do different jobs, but all cells have several things in common. They take in food, digest it, give off waste products, and make new cells.

Every cell has a skinlike covering called a *membrane.* Inside the cell is a syrupy liquid called *cytoplasm.* In the midst of the cytoplasm is a double-walled body that is the cell's control center. It is called the *nucleus,* and it contains the information for creating other cells like itself. The nucleus also has the instructions for making the particular proteins needed for the jobs the cell does.

In the cytoplasm are little bean-shaped energy factories called *mitochondria.* They combine digested food with oxygen to make a special chemical that releases energy when it is broken down. This chemical, *ATP,* is used in the *endoplasmic reticulum,* the cell's protein factory, which is a network of tubes that come out of the *nuclear membrane.* These canals end in the *Golgi bodies,* where the proteins are wrapped, stored, and shipped all over the cell or even outside the cell.

Also within the cytoplasm are fluid-filled sacs called *lysosomes.* They contain enzymes that digest bacteria or injured parts of the cell. When a cell dies, the lysosomes burst and cause the cell to self-destruct.

2

Cell division

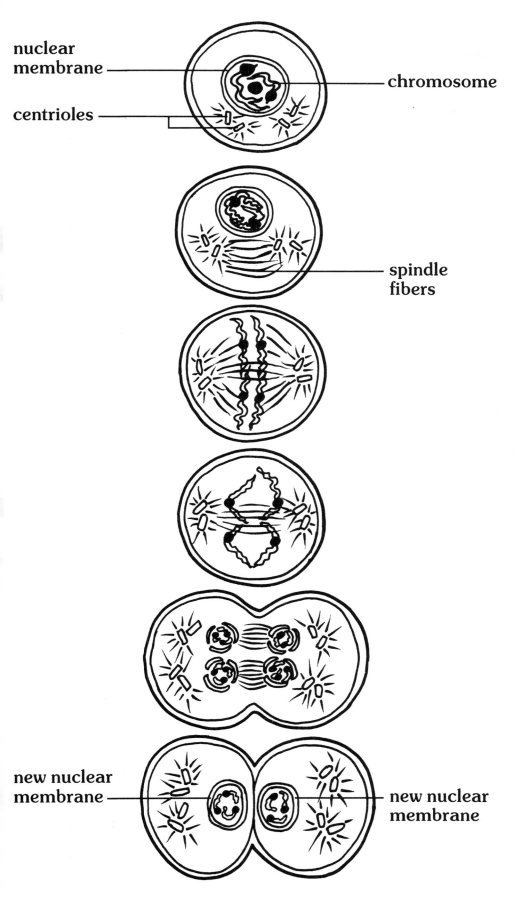

nuclear membrane

centrioles

chromosome

spindle fibers

new nuclear membrane

new nuclear membrane

Cell division All cells can make copies of themselves. This process, called *cell division,* enables the body to grow and to replace worn-out and injured cells.

Directions for cell division are contained in the nucleus of *every* cell. The information is stored on long curly chains of protein called *chromosomes.* Human beings have 46 chromosomes per cell. Each chromosome is made up of many *DNA molecules* and is divided into areas called *genes,* which control different parts of the cell's job.

Cell division always follows the same steps, but it is really one continuous process. First, the *centrioles,* two pairs of tubes outside the nucleus, begin to move to opposite sides of the cell. Between them, tiny microtubes called *spindle fibers* appear. Meanwhile, the chromosomes tighten into cords and copy themselves. Then the membrane, or covering, around the nucleus disappears, and matching chromosomes line up next to each other in pairs. Spindle fibers from each side attach to the chromosomes and pull them apart. The cell membrane begins to pinch inward and new nuclear membranes form around the two chromosome groups. The centrioles copy themselves and the cell membrane pinches through, leaving two separate cells that are identical.

3

The Skeleton

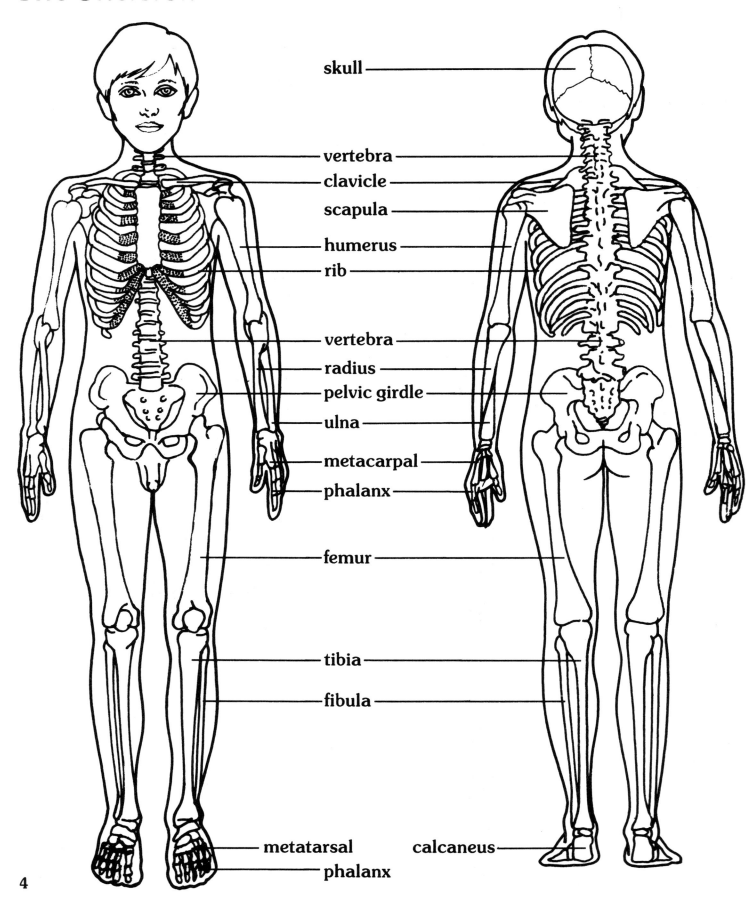

skull

vertebra

clavicle

scapula

humerus

rib

vertebra

radius

pelvic girdle

ulna

metacarpal

phalanx

femur

tibia

fibula

metatarsal

calcaneus

phalanx

The skeleton   There are 206 *bones* in the human body. They give it shape, make it possible to move, protect the organs inside, make blood cells, and store calcium. Bones are alive and continue to replace old cells even after they stop growing and changing shape.

All the bones together are called the *skeleton.* The skeleton has two parts. The *axial skeleton,* the central one, is made up of the skull, the backbone, and the ribs. The *appendicular skeleton,* the outer one, is made up of the arm and leg bones plus the hip and shoulder bones to which they attach.

The legs are attached to the body by the *hipbones,* or *pelvic girdle,* which curve around in a circle, forming a kind of basket that holds and protects the organs in the belly. Between the hip and the knee there is one large bone called the *femur.* Between the knee and the ankle, there are two bones, the *tibia* in front, and the *fibula* to the side. The foot has 26 bones arranged in two arches that help to balance the body and cushion it against shocks.

The arms are attached to the body at the *shoulder girdle,* which is made up of the *collarbone,* or *clavicle,* in front and the *shoulder blade,* or *scapula,* in the back. Between the shoulder and the elbow, there is one big bone called the *humerus.* There are two bones between the elbow and the wrist, the *radius,* which goes to the thumb, and the *ulna,* which ends at the bump on the outside of the wrist. The hand has 27 bones arranged so they can cup, grasp, and pinch.

The skull is made up of several bones that become joined together in the first years of life. The lower jawbone, the *mandible,* is the only movable part of the skull. The *backbone,* or *vertebral column,* is made of 33 neatly stacked bones that hold up the skull. The nerves in the spinal cord run through a hole in the center of the *vertebrae.* The *ribs* attach to the vertebrae in the chest area and curve around to form a cage. All but two ribs attach to the *breastbone,* or *sternum,* in the front. The last nine vertebrae are joined into two bones, the *coccyx* at the tip and, above, the *sacrum,* a shield-shaped bone which attaches to the hips.

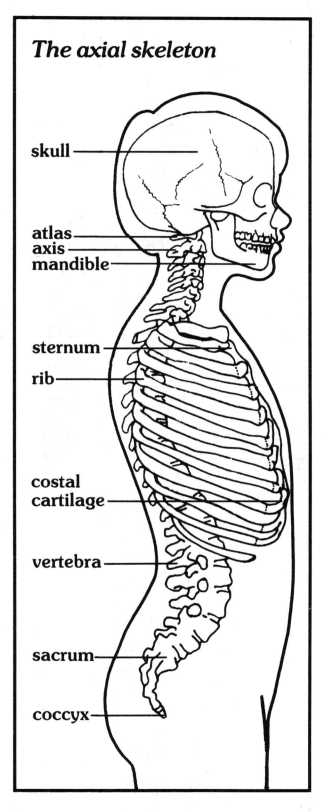

The axial skeleton

skull

atlas
axis
mandible

sternum

rib

costal
cartilage

vertebra

sacrum

coccyx

How bones grow

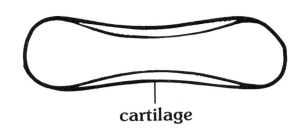

cartilage

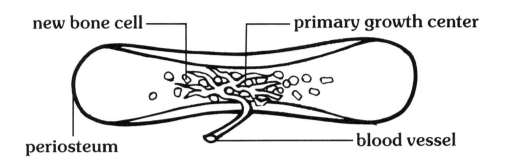

new bone cell — primary growth center

periosteum

blood vessel

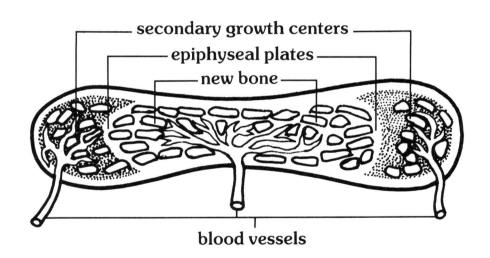

secondary growth centers

epiphyseal plates

new bone

blood vessels

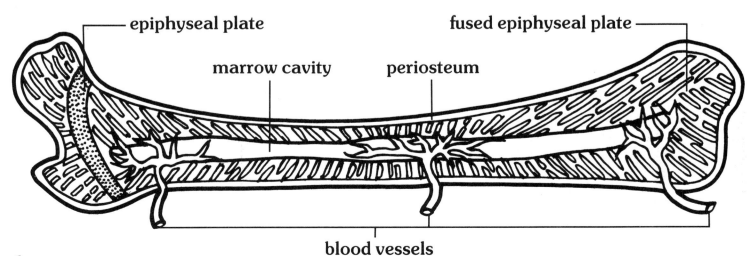

epiphyseal plate

fused epiphyseal plate

marrow cavity

periosteum

blood vessels

How bones grow Bones start forming before birth from a tough rubbery material called *cartilage.* This cartilage model is gradually replaced with bone over a period of years. The process is finished when growth stops.

A *primary growth center* begins to form in the center of the bone. First, tiny crystals of calcium form in the cartilage and make it hard. Next, cartilage cells in the center die off, leaving little holes. Blood vessels from the *periosteum,* the bone covering, grow into these holes. Then cells called *osteoblasts* start to make hard bone, while *osteoclasts* dissolve more tunnels. What forms is a material that looks like a sponge but is hard. A large hollow space called the *marrow cavity* takes shape in the center of the *spongy bone.* Around the outside of the bone, osteoblasts build layers of *compact bone,* which has only microscopic tunnels.

About the time the marrow cavity forms, *secondary growth centers,* like the first one, appear at one end of the bone and then the other. Between the primary and secondary growth centers are flat areas of cartilage called *epiphyseal plates* that continue to grow and lengthen the bone. When the bones reach their full size, the last cartilage cells in the plates die off and are replaced by hard bone. This process, called *fusion,* takes place at different times for different bones and can also vary greatly from one child to another.

The joints The area where two bones meet is called a *joint.* The bones are held together by strong bands called *ligaments* that attach directly to the bones on either side of the joint. Muscles that cross the joint also steady it.

The ends of the bones never actually touch at a joint. They are covered by a layer of rubbery *cartilage,* and they are separated by a tough sac filled with *synovial fluid.* In some joints sliding is made easier by little cartilage pads called *menisci* and little fluid-filled sacs called *bursae.*

Different kinds of joints allow different kinds of movements. The motion a joint can make is determined by the shape of the bones as well as by the location of ligaments and muscles. The hip and shoulder are ball-and-socket joints that move in a circle. The elbow and knee are hinge joints that bend in only one direction. The wrist and ankle are gliding joints that slide up and down. And the skull makes a pivot joint with the top of the backbone.

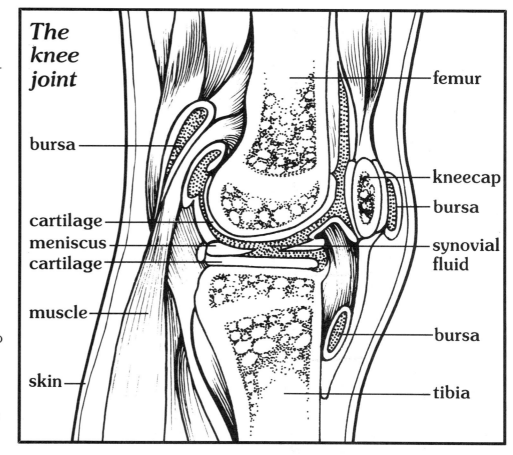

The knee joint

bursa

cartilage
meniscus
cartilage

muscle

skin

femur

kneecap

bursa

synovial fluid

bursa

tibia

The tooth

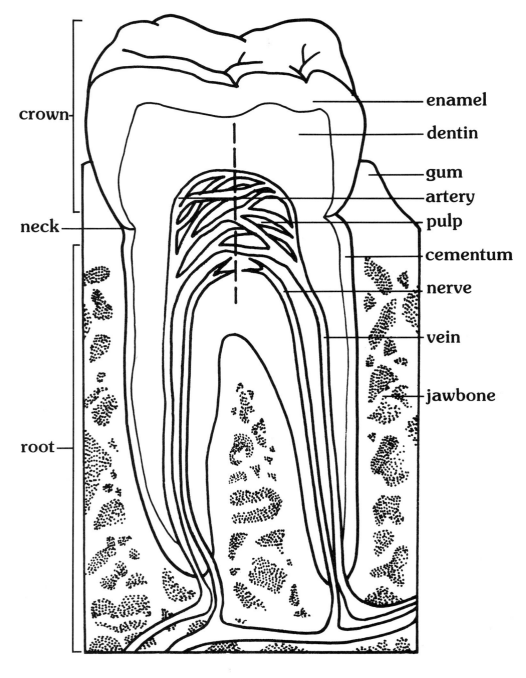

crown

enamel

dentin

neck

gum

artery

pulp

cementum

nerve

vein

jawbone

root

The tooth   The *crown* is the part of the *tooth* you can see above the *gum*, the skin around the tooth. The part of the tooth right at the gum line is called the *neck*. The part under the gum line is called the *root*. It attaches the tooth to the *jawbone*.

All teeth have the same basic structure, but they differ in size, shape, and the number of roots they have. Every tooth is made up of several layers. The *enamel*, the hard part on the outside of the tooth, is made before the tooth comes in. It is nonliving tissue and cannot regrow if a *cavity* makes a hole in it. The enamel is made of calcium and a protein similar to that in hair. It is the hardest substance in the body.

The *dentin* is the layer inside the enamel. It is made of calcium and collagen (like bones). It keeps growing until the tooth dies. In the center of the tooth is the *pulp*. It contains the *nerve* and *blood vessels* in a tube. The pulp brings food and oxygen to the cells in the dentin. The tooth is held in a tight hole in the jawbone, called the *socket*, by *cementum*. The cementum, pulp, and dentin are all living tissues.

age 7

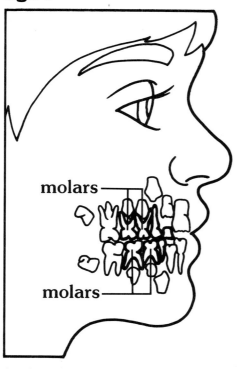

molars
molars

age 9

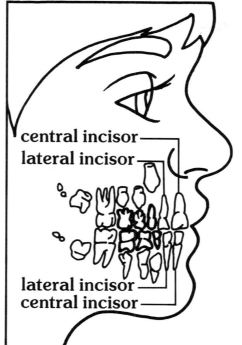

central incisor
lateral incisor

lateral incisor
central incisor

age 11

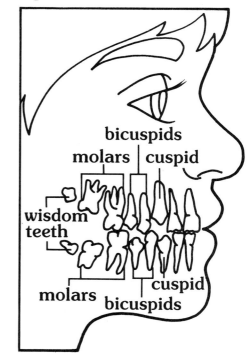

bicuspids
molars | cuspid

wisdom
teeth

molars
bicuspids
cuspid

baby teeth are in darker outline

Tooth eruption   Like most mammals, humans get two sets of teeth. The first set are called *baby,* or *deciduous,* teeth because they naturally fall out during childhood. The second set are called *permanent* teeth because they will last a lifetime if well cared for.

Teeth form completely below the gum but can be seen on an X-ray. The deciduous teeth start to form long before a baby is born. They generally start to *erupt,* or come through the gum, at about six months of age. Over the next year and a half, the 20 baby teeth gradually appear in a fairly set pattern.

There are 32 permanent teeth. They are forming in the gum beneath the baby teeth throughout the early years of childhood. As they push toward the surface, the permanent teeth actually dissolve or erode the roots of the baby teeth, which become wobbly and eventually fall out. Like the baby teeth, the permanent teeth tend to erupt in a fixed sequence, but the exact age at which they appear varies greatly from one child to another. The only rule is that children who

are late getting baby teeth are usually late getting permanent teeth.

The teeth on the upper and lower jaw match. In the front there are two flat *incisors.* On either side of them is a pointed tooth called a *cuspid,* or *eye tooth.* Behind each cuspid are two *bicuspids,* which have two points or cusps. To the rear of these come three pairs of *molars.* They are large flat teeth with several points. The last molars, called the *wisdom teeth,* do not appear in all people. The bicuspids and the last two pairs of molars only appear in the permanent teeth, not in the baby teeth.

The muscles

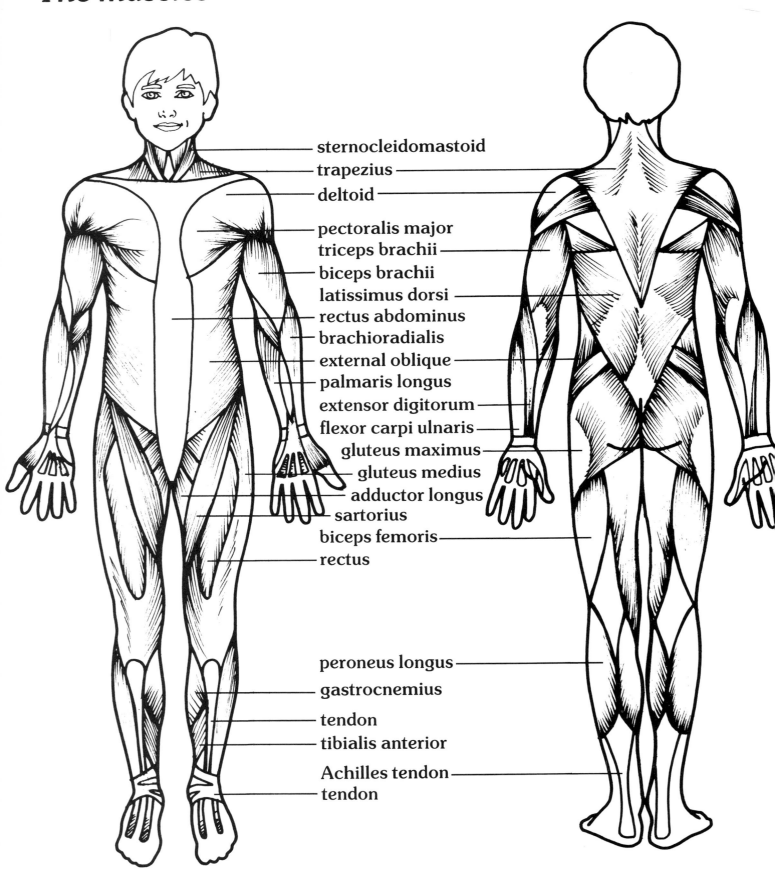

sternocleidomastoid

trapezius

deltoid

pectoralis major
triceps brachii

biceps brachii

latissimus dorsi

rectus abdominus

brachioradialis

external oblique

palmaris longus

extensor digitorum

flexor carpi ulnaris

gluteus maximus

gluteus medius

adductor longus

sartorius

biceps femoris

rectus

peroneus longus

gastrocnemius

tendon

tibialis anterior

Achilles tendon
tendon

The muscles   Humans have 400 different *muscles,* which make up almost half the body. There are three different kinds of muscles, but they all move or contract by alternately squeezing and getting shorter, then relaxing and getting longer. The heart is made of *cardiac muscle.* The blood vessels and digestive system are composed of *smooth muscle.*

The third kind of muscle is the one people usually think of—*skeletal muscle.* All but a few of the skeletal muscles attach to bones at either end with tough bands called *tendons.* When these muscles contract or shorten, they pull one bone toward another. Muscles can only pull; they can't push. So in order to work they are arranged in pairs. One muscle pulls, the other straightens; one turns in, the other turns out. The muscles of the face are unusual because most of them attach to the bottom layer of skin. This is what makes it possible for people to show such a large number of expressions ranging from joy to sadness.

Every skeletal muscle is made up of thousands of elastic *fibers.* A number of fibers make a *bundle;* a number of bundles make a muscle. *Nerves* bring messages from the brain telling different bundles to contract or relax.

Muscles need food and oxygen to work. Also, they get tired if leftover waste products are not taken away by the blood. Very strong people have the same number of fibers in their muscles, but the fibers are bigger because they get more use and their blood supply has been built up. As kids grow, their muscles' fibers become longer and wider. Muscle growth is greatest during the first few years and adolescence.

The muscles of the face

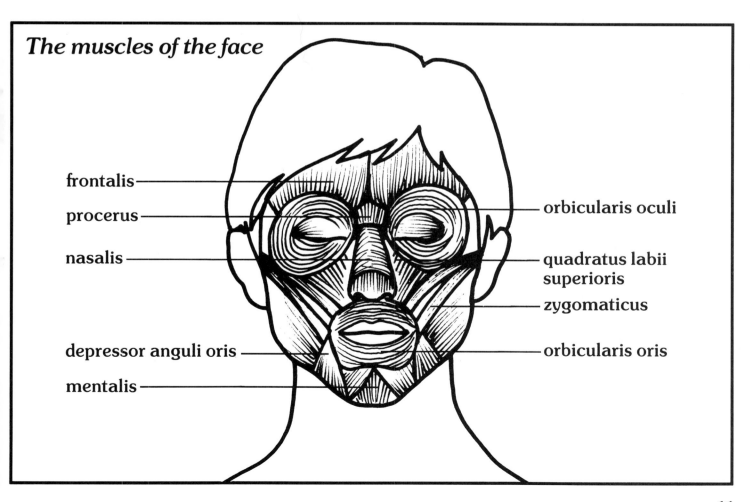

frontalis

procerus

nasalis

depressor anguli oris

mentalis

orbicularis oculi

quadratus labii superioris

zygomaticus

orbicularis oris

How muscles move

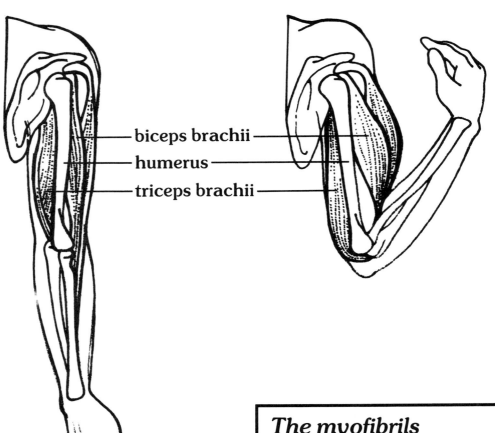

biceps brachii

humerus

triceps brachii

How muscles move Most body movements involve tightening and relaxing opposite groups of muscles. A muscle called the *biceps* attaches to the bones of the forearm and the shoulder. When it contracts, it pulls up the forearm. It gets shorter and fatter and it feels hard. At the same time, the opposing muscle, the *triceps,* relaxes. It gets longer and feels soft. To pull the forearm down, the biceps relaxes and the triceps contracts.

Each muscle fiber is made up of hundreds of thousands of tiny sets of protein bars called *myofibrils.* There are two kinds of bars. One is fat and doesn't move. It has microscopic little arms. The other is thin. When the brain tells a muscle fiber to contract, the little arms pull on the thin bars, which slide in between. In this way the whole muscle becomes shorter and fatter when it contracts.

The myofibrils

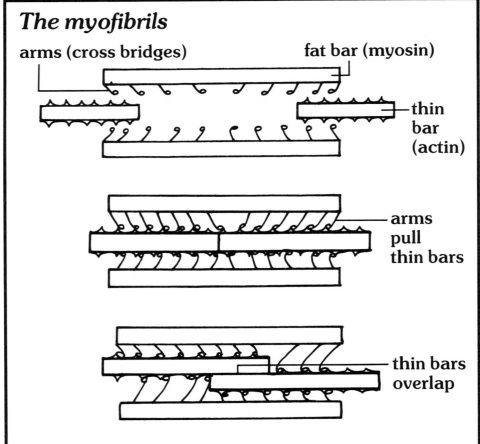

arms (cross bridges)

fat bar (myosin)

thin bar (actin)

arms pull thin bars

thin bars overlap

Temperature regulation

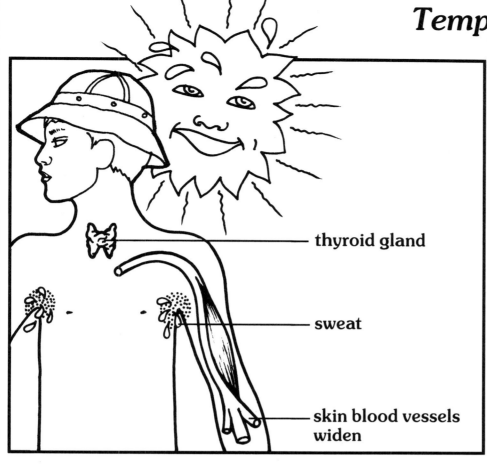

— thyroid gland

— sweat

— skin blood vessels widen

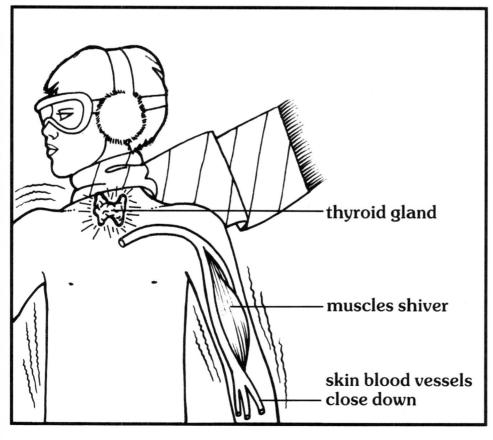

— thyroid gland

— muscles shiver

— skin blood vessels close down

Temperature regulation An area in the center of the brain called the *hypothalamus* controls body temperature. There nerve cells constantly measure the temperature of the nearby blood and send out messages to raise or lower the temperature depending upon whether it's higher or lower than the average 98.6°F, 37°C.

When the body is too warm, the hypothalamus makes three things happen: (1) Blood vessels in the skin are widened, sending up to half the blood to the skin, causing it to radiate heat out into the air; (2) the *thyroid gland* is directed to send out hormones that make cells rest; and (3) the *sweat glands* are put to work pumping out water. As the sweat evaporates it cools the body.

To raise body temperature, the hypothalamus causes the opposite things to happen: (1) It makes blood vessels in the skin squeeze down, sending blood deep into the body; (2) it causes the thyroid gland to send out *hormones* that make the cells take in food and produce more heat; and (3) it makes muscle cells alternately tense and stretch, which causes *shivering*. Shivering makes heat by putting muscle cells to work.

The skin

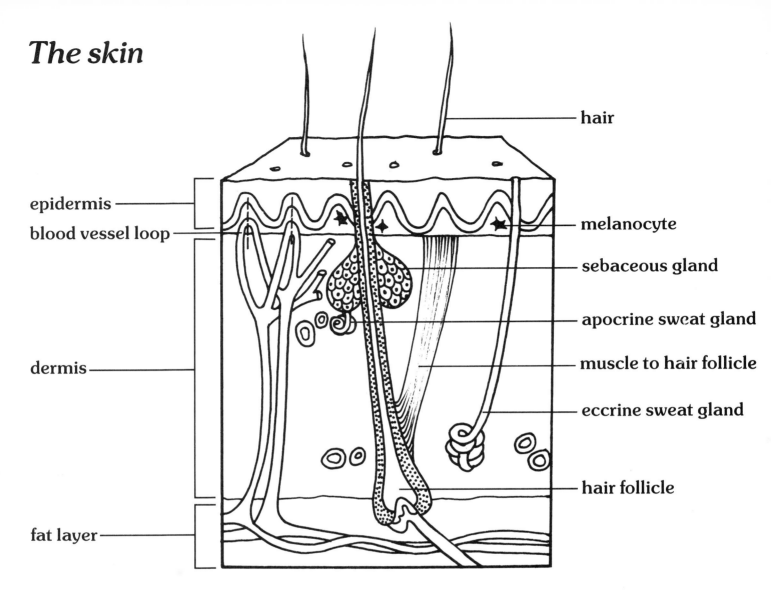

hair

epidermis

blood vessel loop

melanocyte

sebaceous gland

apocrine sweat gland

muscle to hair follicle

eccrine sweat gland

dermis

hair follicle

fat layer

The skin   The *skin* is the body's covering. Its job is to protect the organs and muscles underneath and keep them from drying out. The skin is a barrier that keeps out things like bacteria, but it does let in many chemicals.

The top layer of skin is the *epidermis.* It constantly makes new cells, which gradually harden, die, and fall off. In the bottom of the epidermis are *melanocytes,* cells that give the skin its color and protect it from the sun.

The second layer of skin is called the *dermis.* It is made of cells that are slightly elastic. This layer contains blood vessels, oil glands, sweat glands, hair follicles, and nerves. *Blood vessels* bring food to skin cells and help regulate body temperature. *Hair follicles,* which make the body's hairs, are made of special cells from the epidermis that grow down into the dermis. The *sebaceous glands* make an oily sub-stance that keeps water out and body fluids in. There are two kinds of sweat glands: The *eccrine glands* work when it's hot; the *apocrine glands* begin to work at puberty when people are nervous or excited.

Underneath the dermis is a layer of *fat cells* that cushion the body, store food energy, and insulate the body.

14

Skin messages and the fingernails

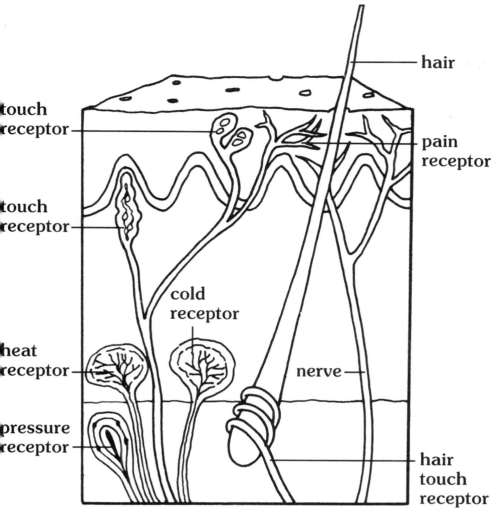

touch receptor

touch receptor

heat receptor

pressure receptor

cold receptor

nerve

hair

pain receptor

hair touch receptor

Skin messages   The skin is not just a covering; it is a sense organ too. "Feeler" nerves in the skin have special endings, or receptors, that send messages to the brain about what is going on outside the body. In the top layer of skin, *pain receptors* signal the brain when the skin is poked by something sharp. There are three kinds of *touch receptors* that signal when something brushes against the skin. *Heat* and *cold receptors* in the middle layer of skin react to outside temperature. In the deepest layer of skin, *pressure receptors* send messages to the brain when something pushes against the body.

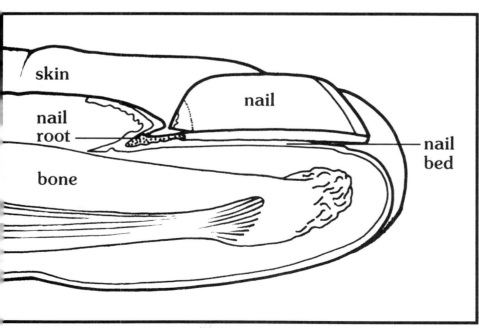

skin

nail

nail root

bone

nail bed

The fingernails   Fingernails and toenails are special areas of the top layer of skin, the *epidermis*. In these areas the cells constantly grow, die, and turn into a hard clear plate. This plate looks pink because of the blood vessels in the skin underneath. Since the cells are dead and there are no nerves in the nails, it doesn't hurt to cut them. Like nails, *hair* comes from a special kind of epidermal cell that dies and can be cut painlessly.

The digestive system

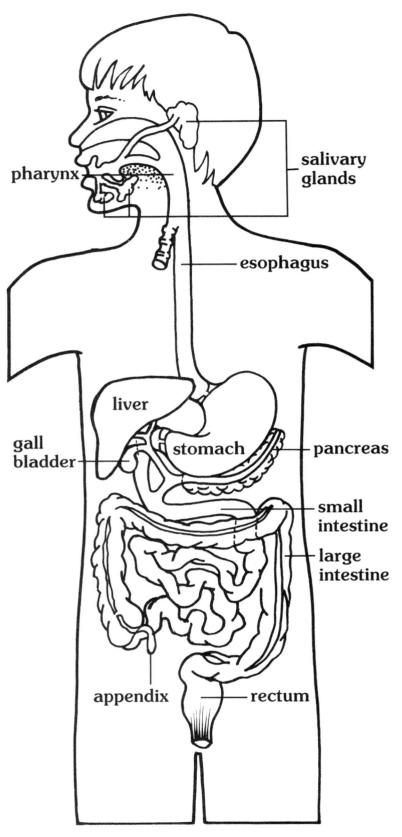

pharynx

salivary glands

esophagus

liver

gall bladder

stomach

pancreas

small intestine

large intestine

appendix

rectum

The digestive system The job of the *digestive system* is to turn food into energy. The system is basically a long tube connected to the outside at both ends and divided into special areas. In each area, substances called *enzymes* break down the food in simpler forms. Finally the food passes into the blood and goes to all parts of the body.

Food enters the mouth and is ground up between the teeth. *Saliva* from three pairs of *salivary glands* moistens the food and starts to break down the carbohydrates in foods like bread and potatoes into simple sugars. Swallowing sends food to the *pharynx*, the back of the throat and down the *esophagus*, a muscular tube that leads to the *stomach*. The stomach has flaps, or *valves*, at either end that keep the food from moving backward.

The stomach is actually a soft muscular bag that can stretch to hold almost a quart of food. Cells in the stomach wall make *hydrochloric acid* and enzymes to dissolve protein and curd milk, and *mucus* to protect the stomach itself from being dissolved. When the food has turned into a thick, milky liquid called *chyme*, it passes on into the *small intestine*. It is here that most of the food is broken down into molecules with the help of three other enzymes. Cells in the wall of the small intestine make *intestinal juice*, cells in the *pancreas*, a small gland behind the stomach, make *pancreatic juice*, and the *liver*, a big organ that lies opposite the stomach, makes *bile*. Bile breaks fats into tiny balls. Intestinal and pancreatic juice further break down fats, proteins, and carbohydrates, which are finally absorbed through the wall of the small intestine into the bloodstream.

What is left over is water, unused enzymes, minerals, and plant fibers called *cellulose*. This mixture passes on into the *large intestine*. The large intestine is the home of millions of healthy bacteria that feed on the fibers and make vitamins B and K. Here minerals needed by the body and most of the water are absorbed. The remaining material, called *feces*, is stored in the *rectum* and later expelled as a bowel movement.

The villi and the liver

The villi   The *villi* are tiny projections that stick out from the walls of the small intestine like the loops of a shaggy carpet. The millions of villi are the places where particles of food are absorbed and put to work in the body. Inside each villus are a connecting *artery* and *vein,* and a little *lymph vessel.* Sugars, minerals, and bits of protein called *amino acids* are carried across the walls of the villi by special chemicals. These food particles enter the villi's blood vessels and are sent to the liver. Fats can enter the bloodstream without any help. They slip into the ends of the lymph vessels in the villi. The fats flow into larger and larger lymph vessels and eventually dump into the bloodstream just above the heart.

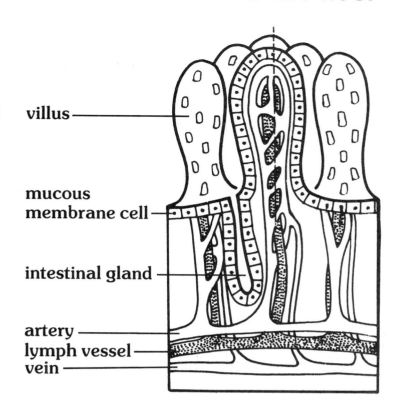

villus

mucous membrane cell

intestinal gland

artery
lymph vessel
vein

The liver   Food particles entering the bloodstream from the small intestine are taken to the *liver* to be further processed. The liver is a large spongelike organ filled with tiny tunnels called *sinusoids.* Blood enters the liver via the *portal vein,* passes through the sinusoids dropping off and picking up food molecules, and leaves through the *hepatic central vein,* which goes to the heart.

Much of the sugar that enters the liver is bundled into long chains called *glycogen* which are stored in the liver until they are needed. The liver also stores amino acids, iron, copper, fat, vitamins A, D, and B_{12} —even extra blood.

In addition to storing extra materials, the liver produces *bile* and many special proteins, including ones necessary for blood clotting and making antibodies. The liver filters alcohol, drugs, and dangerous chemicals out of the blood. They are broken down, attached to bile, sent to the small intestine, and eventually eliminated from the body.

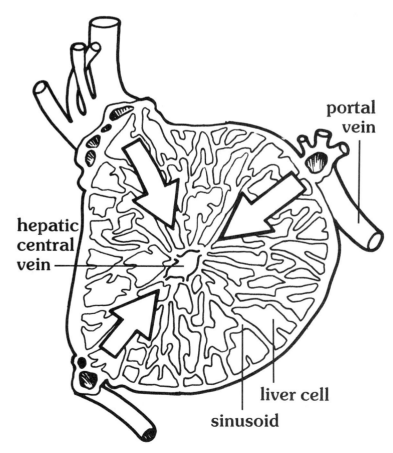

portal vein

hepatic central vein

liver cell

sinusoid

The respiratory system

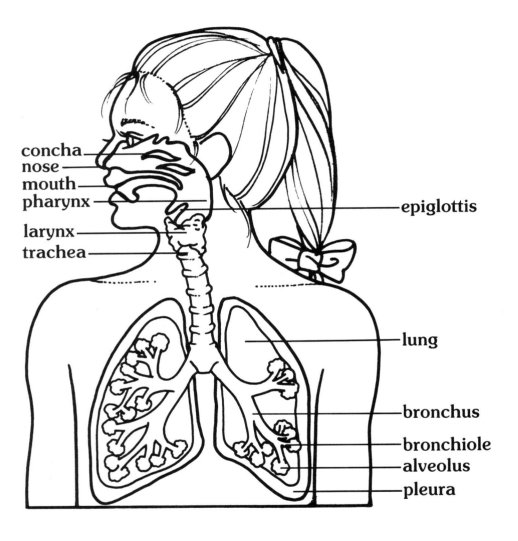

concha
nose
mouth
pharynx

larynx
trachea

epiglottis

lung

bronchus

bronchiole
alveolus
pleura

The respiratory system To stay alive, every cell in the body needs *oxygen* from the air. The job of the *respiratory system* is to get oxygen to the cells and to take away another gas, *carbon dioxide,* that is left over after cells use up the oxygen.

Air enters through the nose or mouth. In the nose it is warmed, moistened, and filtered as it passes over little folds called *con chae.* The nose and mouth join at the back into an area called the *pharynx.* Two tubes open from the bottom of the pharynx: One leads to the stomach and is called the *esophagus;* the other leads to the *lungs* and is called the *windpipe,* or *trachea.* At the top of the windpipe is the *voice box,* or *larynx.* It is covered by a little flap named the *epiglottis.* This flap closes over the windpipe during swallowing and prevents food from entering the lungs.

The windpipe is made of many C-shaped cartilage rings with a tough elastic covering. In the chest the windpipe splits into two branches called the *bronchi* —one for each lung—which divide into smaller and smaller tubes called the *bronchioles.* Every tiny tube ends in a little sac called an *alveolus,* or *air sac.* The lungs are each covered with a membrane called the *pleura.*

The vocal cords and the cilia

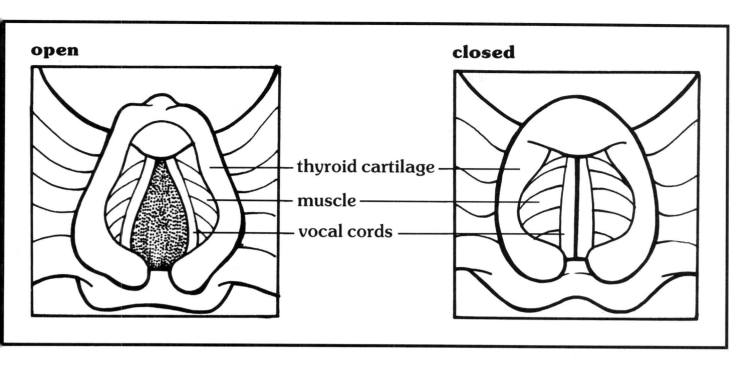

open   closed

thyroid cartilage

muscle

vocal cords

The vocal cords The *voice box,* or *larynx,* sits at the top of the windpipe. It is triangle shaped and sticks out from the neck in a bump called the *Adam's apple.*

Inside the voice box are two elastic bands called the *vocal cords.* They help to control what goes into the lungs, and they make speech possible. When people breathe in or out, the vocal cords are open. When people swallow food, the cords are closed. When people talk, the vocal cords are almost closed. As air passes over them, they vibrate and make a noise. When people cough, the vocal cords close until pressure builds, then they blast

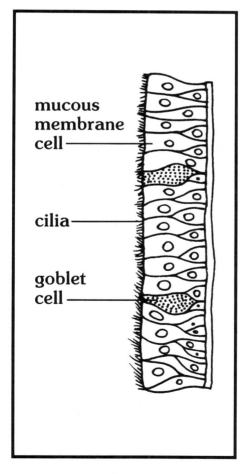

mucous membrane cell

cilia

goblet cell

open as air rushes out of the lungs at up to 70 miles an hour. This blast of air can help to clear the throat of dirt, phlegm, or food.

The cilia The nose and throat are lined with special cells. Their job is to keep the lungs clear of dirt and food particles that could plug up the tiny air sacs. *Goblet cells* make a watery fluid called *mucus.* Dirt particles that enter the throat stick to the mucus. The particles are then moved along by millions of tiny arms called *cilia* that stick out from the cells lining the throat.

Breathing in and out

inhaling

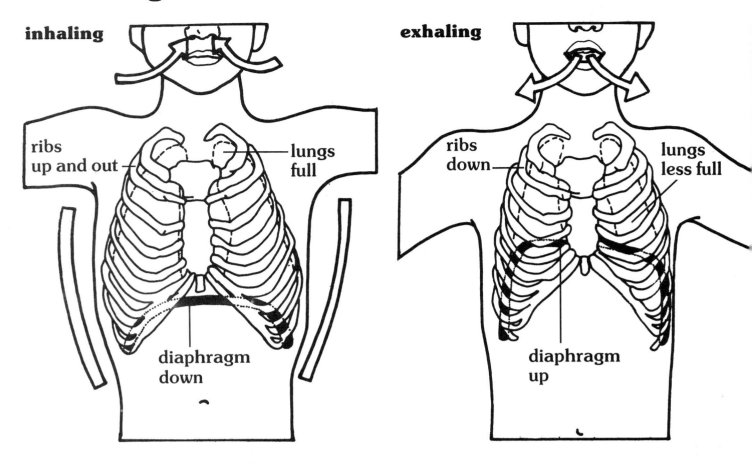

ribs
up and out

lungs
full

diaphragm
down

exhaling

ribs
down

lungs
less full

diaphragm
up

Breathing in and out Breathing brings air into and out of the lungs. Bringing air into the lungs is called *inhaling*. Sending air out of the lungs is called *exhaling*.

The lungs do not breathe by themselves: They are elastic and can stretch, but they have no muscles. Air is moved by the muscles of the ribs and a great thick muscle called the *diaphragm*. It sits under the lungs and separates the chest compart-ment from the belly. The diaphragm does three-quarters of the work of breathing, and the rib muscles do one-quarter.

When people breathe in, the diaphragm tightens, flattens, and drops. This pulls down the lungs and makes the chest compart-ment longer. At the same time, the muscles between the ribs tighten. This raises the ribs and makes the chest compartment wider. Since the chest compart-ment is sealed, a vacuum forms and air is sucked in. After people breathe in, the diaphragm and rib muscles relax. The chest falls back the way it was, the dia-phragm goes back up, and air is pushed out of the lungs.

Even though people can change their breathing on pur-pose, most of the time they breathe automatically. Automati breathing is controlled by a spe-cial center in the lower brain called the *medulla*. Kids usually breathe about 20 times a minute When they exercise, they breath much faster because the body needs more oxygen.

How air gets into the blood

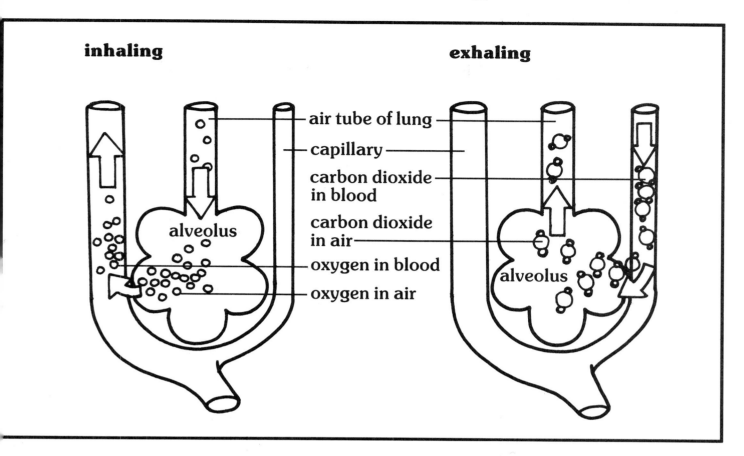

inhaling

exhaling

air tube of lung

capillary

carbon dioxide in blood

carbon dioxide in air

oxygen in blood

oxygen in air

alveolus

alveolus

How air gets into the blood
The lungs contain three million *air sacs,* or *alveoli.* Their job is to get oxygen into the blood and to remove *carbon dioxide,* a gas left over after cells do their work.

Every air sac is surrounded by tiny blood vessels called *capillaries. Red blood cells* come into these capillaries carrying molecules of carbon dioxide. The carbon dioxide passes through the wall of the air sac and is exhaled from the lungs.

Meanwhile, oxygen molecules in the air sac enter the bloodstream and are picked up by the red blood cells that have just gotten rid of their carbon dioxide load. These red blood cells pass through the *heart* and carry oxygen to all parts of the body.

Each red blood cell can carry millions of molecules of oxygen or carbon dioxide. The respiratory center in the brain that controls breathing is set so that the amount of carbon dioxide in the blood never goes above a certain level. People whose lungs have been damaged by smoking or dirt have to breathe more often to get the same amount of oxygen as people with healthy lungs.

The circulatory system

The circulatory system The *circulatory system* is a giant network of tubes that carries the *blood* from the *heart* out to the body and back to the heart. The heart itself is a big pump that pushes the blood out to the body. The circulatory system actually makes two loops, or circles. First it goes to the lungs and back, then it goes to the body and back. On the loop to the body, the blood drops off oxygen and food; it returns with carbon dioxide and other waste products. Food is picked up in the liver, oxygen in the lungs. Carbon dioxide is dropped off in the lungs, the other waste products in the *kidneys*. The blood also transports hormones from the brain and the glands to other organs and cells.

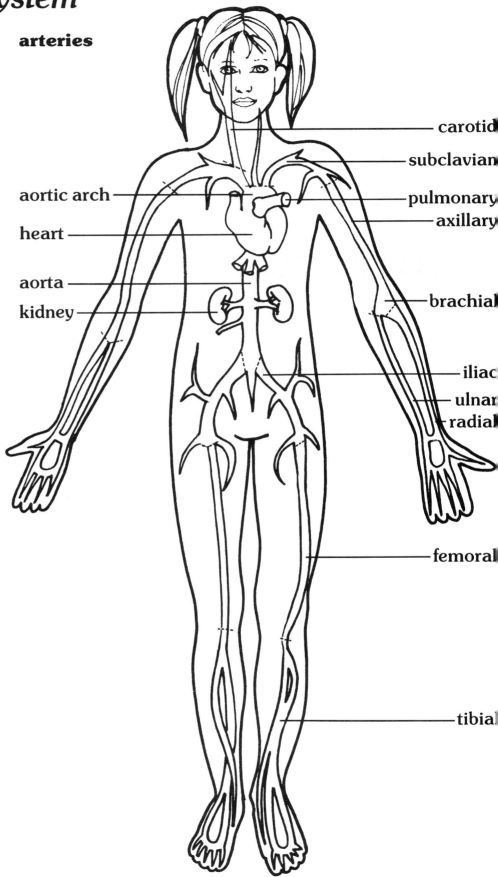

arteries

carotid

subclavian

pulmonary

axillary

aortic arch

heart

brachial

aorta

kidney

iliac

ulnar

radial

femoral

tibial

22

Arteries and veins

veins

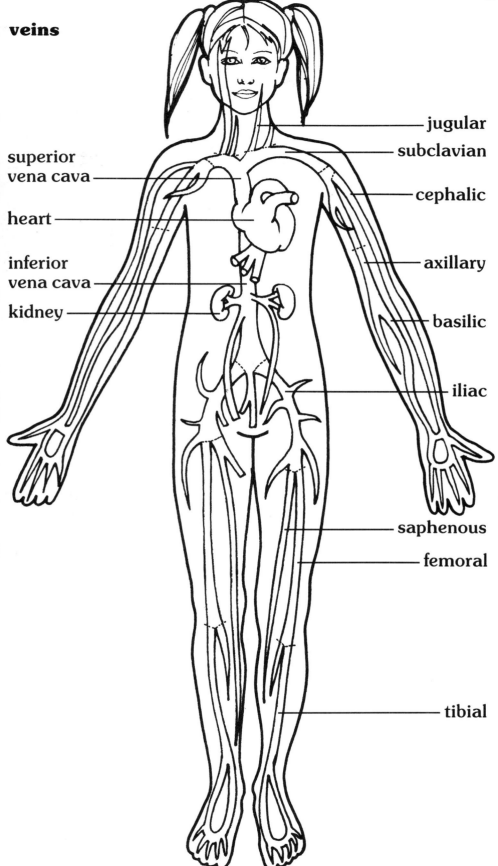

jugular

subclavian

superior vena cava

cephalic

heart

axillary

inferior vena cava

kidney

basilic

iliac

saphenous

femoral

tibial

Arteries and veins The biggest blood vessels carrying blood out to the body are called *arteries*. Major arteries go to the head, the arms, the lungs, the abdomen, and even to the heart itself. These arteries branch into smaller and smaller tubes. The smallest arteries form a loop, or net, with the smallest veins.

The *veins* are the tubes that carry blood back to the heart after it has dropped off its food and oxygen. Large veins run near the large arteries from all the major parts of the body.

Artery walls have both elastic and muscular fibers. Every time the heart beats and pumps blood into the arteries, they stretch a little. Between beats they shrink back but don't flatten out because of their muscle fibers. By the time the blood reaches the veins, it no longer is pushed by the pressure of the heart beating. In fact, the veins have tiny valves like one-way doors to keep the blood from flowing backward. The contraction of nearby muscles squeezes the veins and helps to push the blood back to the heart.

The capillaries and blood composition

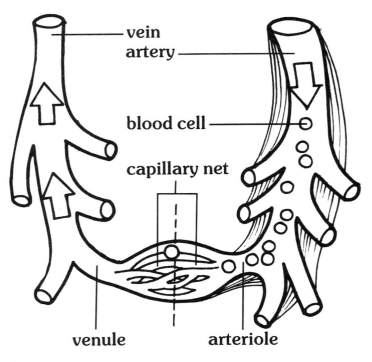

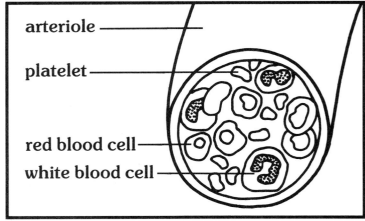

The capillaries and blood composition   The tiniest blood vessels in the body are microscopic. They are called the *capillaries*. Here arteries and veins join in a net, and outgoing blood finishes its journey and begins its return to the heart.

Blood reaches the capillaries carrying molecules of food and oxygen. These molecules slip out to the cells through very tiny holes in the walls of the capillaries. Meanwhile, carbon dioxide and molecules the body needs to get rid of enter the holes and are carried off by the blood returning to the heart. Carbon dioxide is eventually dropped off in the lungs, the other wastes in the kidneys.

In some parts of the body, the capillaries do other jobs as well. In the lungs, capillary nets exchange carbon dioxide and oxygen. In the kidneys, the capillaries filter out waste products; in the small intestine, they pick up food that the digestive system has broken down to molecule-size particles; and in the glands, they pick up hormones that are eventually dropped off all over the body.

The blood is made up of about half cells, half water, and a small amount of proteins and mineral salts. The minerals include calcium, iron, magnesium, sodium, and zinc. Blood without cells is called *plasma*. It is a yellow fluid made up of water and dissolved substances including food, vitamins, hormones, antibodies, waste products, oxygen, and carbon dioxide.

Almost all the cells in the blood are *red blood cells*. Each red blood cell can carry millions of molecules of oxygen or carbon dioxide. These cells look like flat red Frisbees. Actually they are elastic bags that can twist into strange shapes but cannot fit through the tiny holes in the walls of the capillaries. Each drop of blood has half a million red blood cells.

The second kind of cell in the blood is the *white blood cell*. There are two basic types of white blood cells: One kind eats germs, the other makes antibodies that can "lock up" germs. White blood cells are much bigger than the red blood cells, but they are able to squeeze through the holes in the capillaries and get out to the cells. Other white cells live permanently in the liver, lungs, and lymph nodes. Generally there are only 150 white blood cells per drop of blood. When the body is sick or has an infection, it can make four times that many in a few hours.

The third kind of blood cell is *platelets*. They are tiny pieces broken off of big cells in the bone marrow. Platelets are sticky and they help to form blood clots.

How the heart pumps

How the heart pumps   The heart is a hollow muscle shaped like a pine cone. It is located near the middle of the chest, between the right and left lungs. The heart's job is to pump the blood, first to the lungs and then to the rest of the body. To do this the heart is divided down the middle into two pumps that are separate but work at the same time. Each pump has two parts, or chambers: The top chambers are called the *atria,* the bottom chambers are called the *ventricles.* Each of the four chambers is actually a little pump in itself. Blood enters both top chambers at the same time. The left atrium gets blood with fresh oxygen from the lungs; the right atrium gets blood with carbon dioxide from the body. Then the atria squeeze and fill the ventricles. Next both ventricles squeeze at the same time. The right ventricle sends the blood loaded with carbon dioxide to the lungs; the left sends oxygen-rich blood to the body. Between the heart's chambers are *valves,* little flaps that act like one-way doors and keep blood from going backward. When pushed hard enough from the inside, they open. If pushed from the wrong side, they close tighter.

The pumping of the chambers happens very quickly and produces one *beat,* or *stroke,* of the heart, after which the heart rests for a longer time. Each heartbeat is started by a special group of cells at the top of the heart called the *pacemaker.* They tighten first, and then the contraction spreads like a wave from the top to the bottom of the heart. This is what makes the top chambers squeeze a little ahead of the lower chambers. The heart beats about 75 times a minute in women and about 65 times in men. At birth the average heart rate is 130 to 135. This rate drops to almost the adult rate by ten years.

Suggestion:

Color the blood on the left side of the heart red, and the blood on the right side blue.

blood in atria

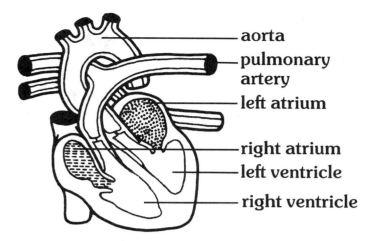

- aorta
- pulmonary artery
- left atrium
- right atrium
- left ventricle
- right ventricle

blood in ventricles

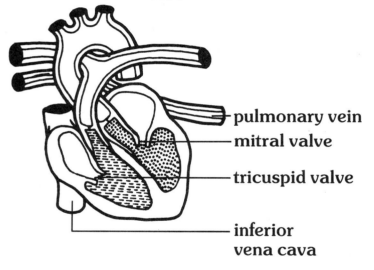

- pulmonary vein
- mitral valve
- tricuspid valve
- inferior vena cava

blood to arteries and lungs

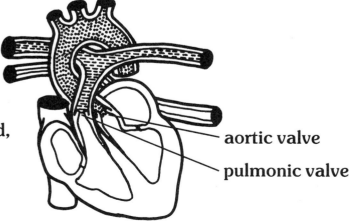

- aortic valve
- pulmonic valve

25

The lymph system

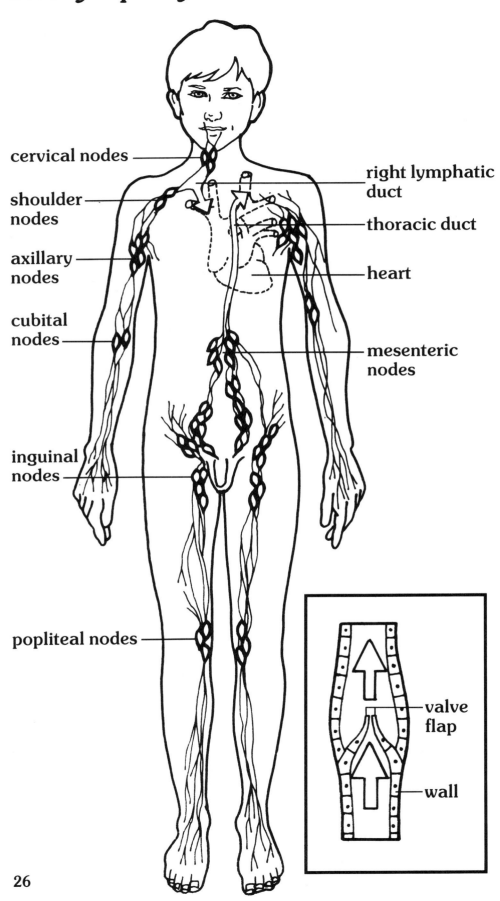

cervical nodes

shoulder nodes

axillary nodes

cubital nodes

inguinal nodes

popliteal nodes

right lymphatic duct

thoracic duct

heart

mesenteric nodes

valve flap

wall

The lymph system   All the cells in the body are surrounded by fluid that carries food and oxygen molecules from the blood vessels to the cells and brings back waste products. Most extra fluid and protein molecules return to the blood vessels, but some do not. The job of the lymph system is to take away this extra fluid, which is called *lymph,* and keep the body from swelling up.

The lymph system is like a giant network of one-way drains. They start out small and lead into bigger and bigger tubes called *lymphatic vessels.* After all the vessels join together, they dump into one of the largest blood vessels entering the heart.

When lymph starts building up around the cells, pressure grows, and the fluid and proteins seep into holes in the walls of the smallest lymph vessels. Little flaps called *valves* keep the fluid from flowing backward, and when the muscles near the lymph vessels contract, they push the fluid along.

Lymph vessels pass through filters called *lymph nodes.* There are grapelike clusters of these nodes in the major areas that the lymph system drains: the neck, elbow, armpit, shoulder, knee, crotch, and abdomen.

How a lymph node works

How a lymph node works

Lymph enters a node from the lymphatic vessels and flows into little areas called *sinuses,* which are filled with a fine net of fibers. This net lets the fluid pass but traps bacteria, viruses, and poisons. Special white blood cells called *macrophages* live in the area called the *medulla.* The macrophages surround and eat trapped substances and spit out leftover proteins. This process is called *phagocytosis.*

In another part of the node, called the *cortex,* the leftover proteins are used to identify and fight the dangerous substances. A different kind of white blood cell, called a *lymphocyte,* lives in the cortex. These cells make a special *antibody* to lock around the dangerous protein, or *antigen.* Once the lymphocyte has learned to do this, it divides over and over again, making hundreds of cells like itself, and sends them all over the body to hunt for that kind of germ. When a person is sick, the lymph nodes become very active filtering out substances and making antibodies to fight them. During the active time, the nodes in that area of the body temporarily become big and swollen and can even be painful.

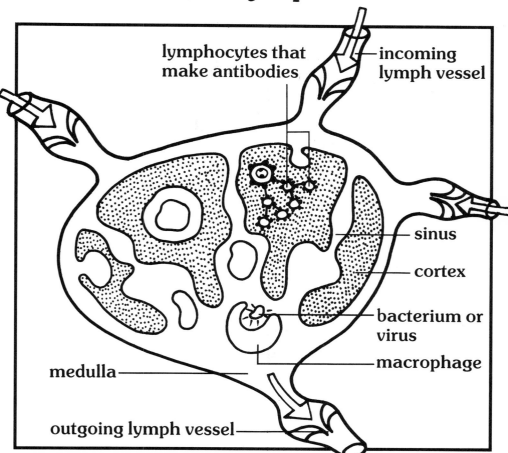

lymphocytes that make antibodies

incoming lymph vessel

sinus

cortex

bacterium or virus

macrophage

medulla

outgoing lymph vessel

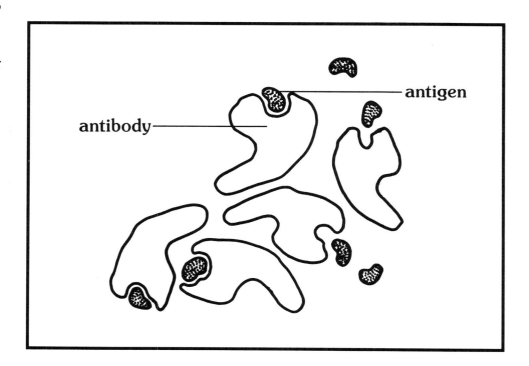

antigen

antibody

The urinary system

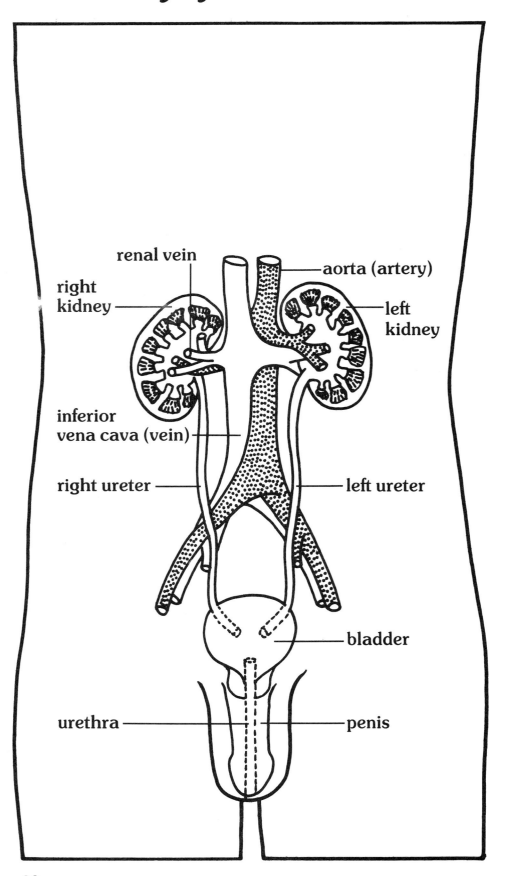

renal vein

aorta (artery)

right kidney

left kidney

inferior vena cava (vein)

right ureter

left ureter

bladder

urethra

penis

The urinary system Every cell in the body contains fluid and is surrounded by fluid containing water, salt, minerals, and waste products left over from cell work. For cells to remain alive, the wastes have to be taken away, and there has to be the right amount of salt and other minerals. This is the job of the *urinary system.* Excess minerals and waste products enter the bloodstream and are carried to the *kidneys.* The kidneys are two bean-shaped organs that lie behind the belly button close to the backbone. It is the kidneys' job to filter the blood to remove waste products, water, and, if necessary, minerals. The fluid that is filtered out is called *urine.* The urine passes from the kidneys into the *ureters,* ten-inch muscular tubes that squeeze it into the *bladder,* a muscular bag that sits at the bottom of the abdomen where the legs join the body. The bladder has many folds in its sides, so it can stretch to hold as much as two cups of urine. At the bottom of the bladder is a ring-shaped muscle called a *sphincter.* When the sphincter is closed, the bladder stores urine. When a person urinates, the sphincter opens. Then the urine passes into the *urethra,* a tube that leads to outside the body. In girls the urethra is short and comes out just above the vagina. In boys the urethra is longer and passes down through the penis.

How the kidney works Each kidney contains a million *nephrons,* which work to filter out waste products from the blood and turn them into urine. Making urine is a two-step process. First, several products are removed in a part of the nephron called the *glomerulus.* Then, in the nephron's *tubule,* certain substances are returned to the bloodstream in the exact amounts the body needs.

The glomerulus is a microscopic pressurized filter made of tiny blood vessels with holes in their walls. Water, minerals, salts, and wastes are pushed through the holes into the tubule. The tubule runs out from the glomerulus, turns sharply at the *loop of Henle,* and runs back up into a central *collecting tube* that sends the urine on to the bladder. Wrapped around each tubule is a blood vessel that comes from the glomerulus and leads out of the kidney. At the top of the tubule, sugar and vitamins are actively transported back into the blood vessel. In the loop, most of the water and whatever salt the body needs are absorbed back into the blood. Every day about 180 quarts of liquid are filtered out; all but about one quart passes back into the blood. Otherwise the body would become totally dried out within a few hours.

the nephron

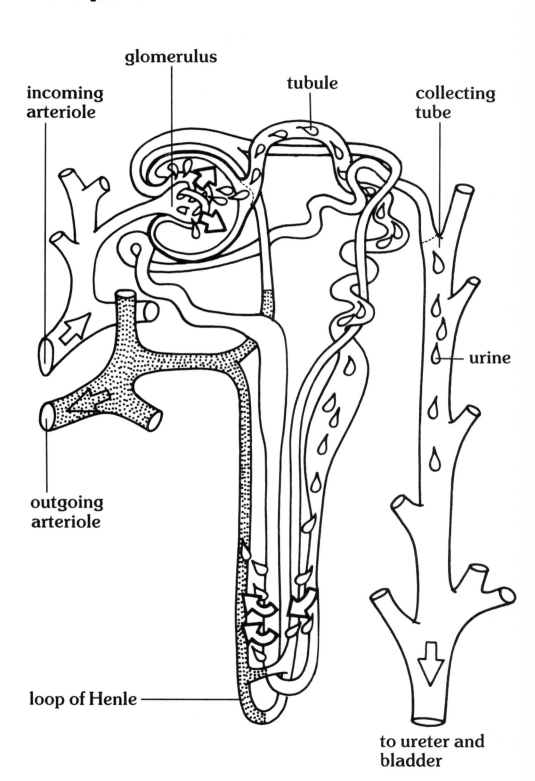

glomerulus

incoming arteriole

tubule

collecting tube

urine

outgoing arteriole

loop of Henle

to ureter and bladder

The nervous system

The nervous system   The *nervous system* is a complicated network of 12 billion cells that links all parts of the body so they can work together. The system has three kinds of cells: "feelers," "thinkers," and "doers." *Sensory nerve cells* are designed to "feel." They tell the body what's going on. Outside they report on sound, smell, taste, sight, skin temperature, touch, and pain. Inside they report on body position, body temperature, blood pressure, pain, and blood levels of oxygen, waste products, hormones, and so on.

Incoming messages are sent to "thinkers," *integrative nerve cells,* who decide what messages mean and what the body should do. They send messages to *motor nerve cells,* "doers," who make glands and organs work and muscles move.

The integrative cells, or thinkers, are located in the *spinal cord* and the *brain.* They make up the *central nervous system.* The sensory and motor cells, the feelers and the doers, are located all over the body. They make up the *peripheral,* or *outer, nervous system.*

Nerves consist of many cells bundled in a tough covering. Sensory and motor cells lie side by side within this sheath, but they are wrapped in a fatty layer that keeps messages separate.

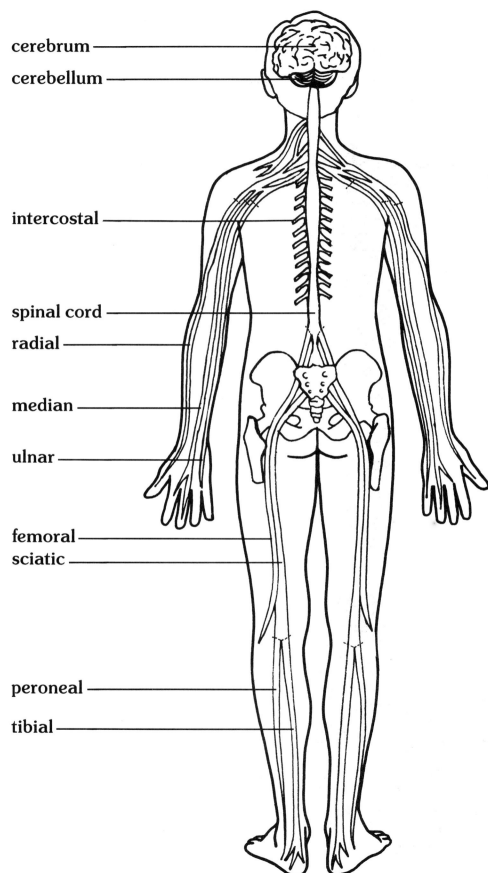

cerebrum

cerebellum

intercostal

spinal cord

radial

median

ulnar

femoral

sciatic

peroneal

tibial

The brain and the spinal cord
The nerves in the spinal cord are arranged in bundles, or *tracts*, based on what they do. There are matching tracts for each side of the body, and each tract carries just one kind of motor or sensory nerve. In the brain, thinker, or integrative, cells are arranged into groups, or areas, based on what they do. Their jobs get more complicated and less automatic the higher the cells are located in the brain.

The *medulla* and the *pons* at the bottom of the brain have control of many of the automatic functions that keep people alive: breathing, heartbeat, blood pressure, swallowing, and digestion. The *cerebellum* controls balance and helps groups of muscles work together smoothly without thought.

The big, thinking part of the brain is called the *cerebrum*. It contains areas that store memories, receive and sort out sensory information, and control *endocrine glands*, emotions, and body movements. Each side of the cerebrum controls somewhat different functions. The *left side* thinks about words, numbers, and putting things in order. The *right side* keeps track of where all parts of the body are in space and flashes on ideas or solutions to problems.

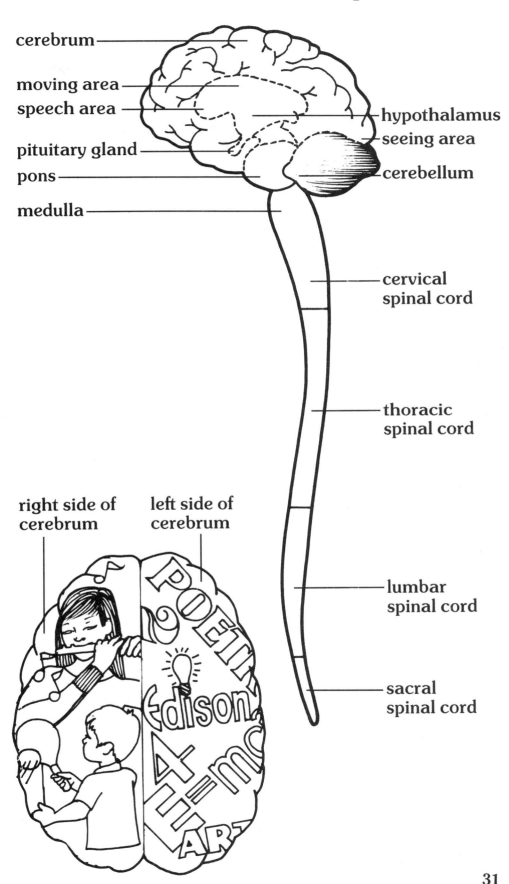

cerebrum

moving area

speech area

pituitary gland

pons

medulla

hypothalamus

seeing area

cerebellum

cervical spinal cord

thoracic spinal cord

lumbar spinal cord

sacral spinal cord

right side of cerebrum

left side of cerebrum

31

Reflexes

Reflexes The whole nervous system works by combining the jobs of the three kinds of nerve cells—the feelers, thinkers, and doers—in a chain, or circuit. The simplest circuits are called *reflexes*. They don't require a person to think; they happen automatically. For example, reflexes control breathing, heartbeat, and balance. The thinker cells in a reflex chain are in the spinal cord or the lower brain, not in the cerebrum.

One of the simplest reflexes is the knee-jerk. Just below the knee there are feeler nerve cells that measure the tension in the big thigh muscle. If these cells are tapped, they alert doer cells that tighten the muscle more and cause the foot to swing forward automatically. Most other reflexes use a thinker cell in the spinal cord to figure out the message.

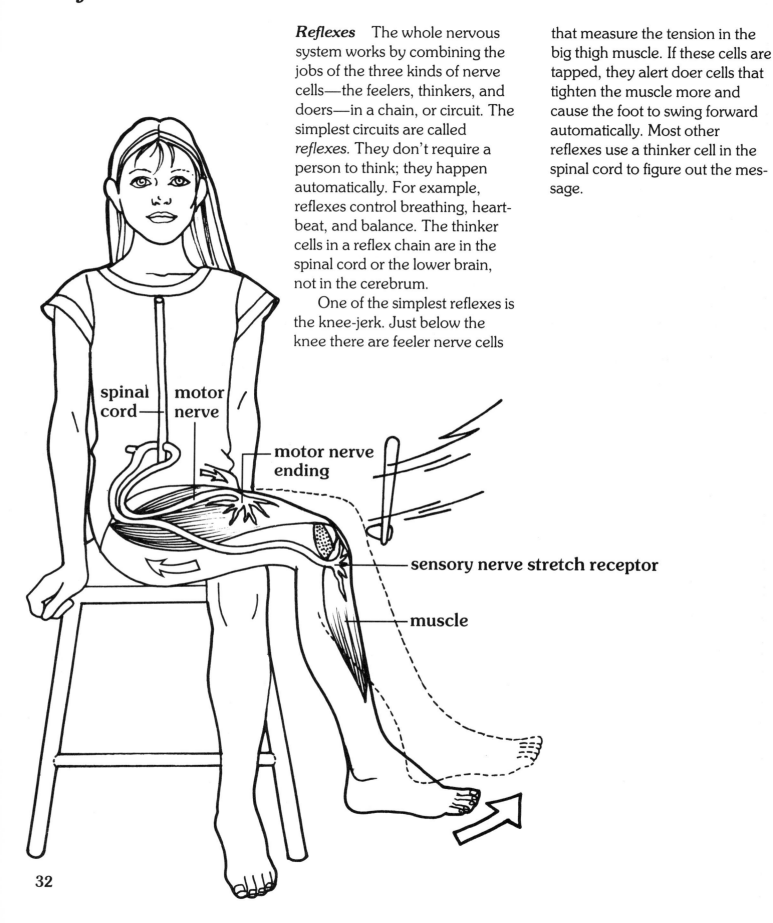

spinal cord

motor nerve

motor nerve ending

sensory nerve stretch receptor

muscle

The nerve cell and the synapse

The nerve cell   Every nerve cell has three basic parts: a body and an incoming and outgoing arm. The body contains the *nucleus,* the control center for the cell. The incoming arm, called the *dendrite,* brings in messages. A nerve cell can have a number of dendrites coming from different places. But there is never more than one outgoing arm. It is called the *axon,* and it carries messages to the next cell.

All nerve signals travel in only one direction. The nervous system is like a map with only one-way streets. Each nerve signal is a tiny burst of electricity that travels in along the dendrite, across the body, and out the axon in a fraction of a second.

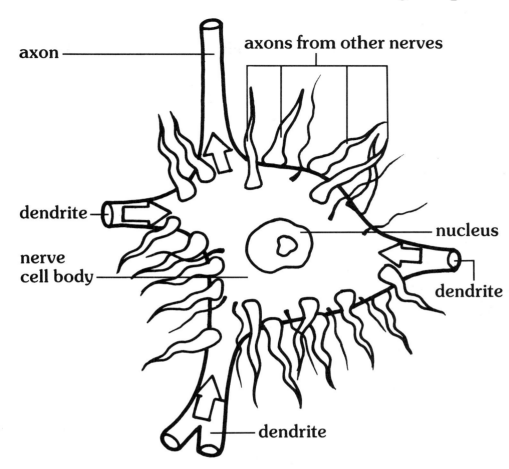

The synapse   The axon of one nerve cell never actually touches another nerve cell. They are always separated by a small space called the *synapse.* The electrical message carried along one nerve cell cannot jump to the next. Instead the *bulb,* or bump, at the end of the axon releases little chemical sacs that cross the synapse. When enough sacs touch the dendrite of the next cell, the message passes down it. Thus the synapse, like the nerve cell itself, works in only one direction.

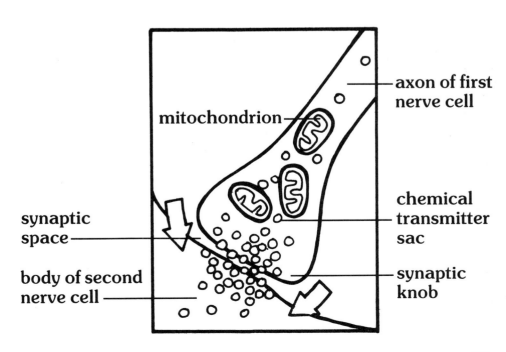

The autonomic nervous system

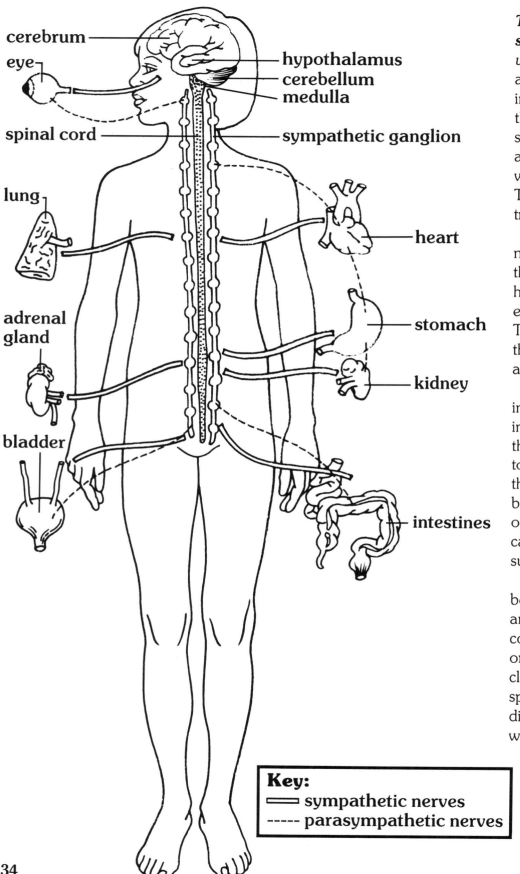

cerebrum

eye

hypothalamus

cerebellum

medulla

spinal cord

sympathetic ganglion

lung

heart

adrenal gland

stomach

kidney

bladder

intestines

Key:

⬜ sympathetic nerves

----- parasympathetic nerves

The autonomic nervous system The *autonomic nervous system* takes care of the automatic functions, like breathing and digestion, that we don't think about. To do this it constantly checks the body's organs and glands and keeps them working at just the right speed. The brain's *hypothalamus* controls these functions.

The system has two kinds of nerves that basically do opposite things. The *sympathetic nerves* help the body prepare for action, especially in times of emergency. The *parasympathetic nerves* help the body slow down, digest food, and repair itself.

The sympathetic nerves start in the spinal cord and pass out into the *ganglia* on either side of the spinal cord, and continue on to different organs. They make the heart beat faster, send more blood to the lungs and muscles, open up lung passages, and cause the liver to send out more sugar for extra energy.

The parasympathetic nerves begin at the bottom of the brain and the bottom of the spinal cord. They go directly to different organs. They slow the heart, close down lung passages, and speed up digestion. They also direct the muscles that control when people go to the bathroom.

The eye

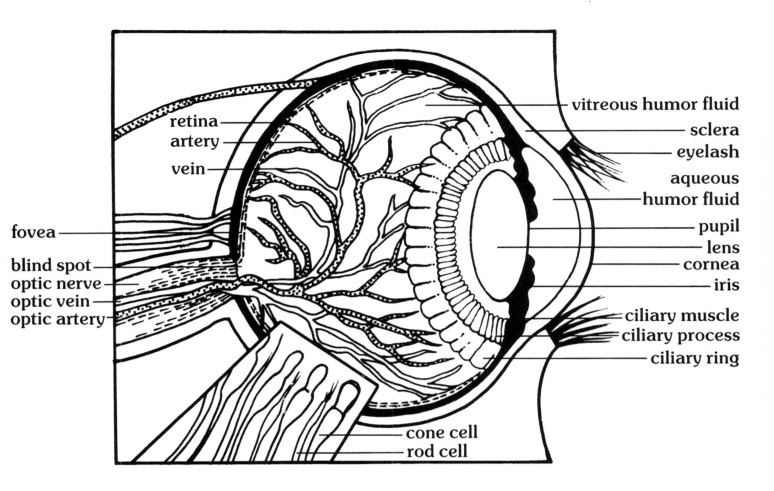

retina
artery
vein

fovea

blind spot
optic nerve
optic vein
optic artery

vitreous humor fluid
sclera
eyelash
aqueous
humor fluid
pupil
lens
cornea
iris
ciliary muscle
ciliary process
ciliary ring

cone cell
rod cell

The eye The *eye* is a special part of the nervous system. The back of the *eye*, the *retina*, is lined with "feeler" cells. It is their job to pick up light and send messages along the *optic nerve* to the brain.

The eye is a hollow ball made of tough white fibers. This ball, called the *sclera*, is packed with a clear, thick fluid called the *vitreous humor*. In front of this fluid is the *lens*, a rubbery disk that focuses incoming light on the retina. A ring called the *ciliary muscle* circles the lens and adjusts its focus. In front of the lens is another muscular ring, the *iris*,

which is the colored part of the eye. It controls how much light gets into the eye. The black hole in the center of the iris is called the *pupil.* The front of the sclera, called the *cornea,* is clear. It focuses light on the lens, but it cannot be adjusted. Between the cornea and the lens is another fluid-filled area called the *aqueous humor.* It brings food and oxygen to the cornea.

The retina contains two types of light-sensing cells: *rods* and *cones.* Most of the cells are rods.

They pick up low amounts of light, work well in dark situations, and provide a general picture. Most of the cones are located in the middle of the retina in an area called the *fovea.* The cones work best in bright light, provide a sharp picture, and are responsible for color vision. There are three types of cone cells—red, blue, and green. Colors that are mixtures excite more than one kind of cone cell. There is one place on the retina, called the *blind spot,* that has no light-sensing cells because the arms of the rods and cones come together to form the optic nerve.

The eye muscles and tears

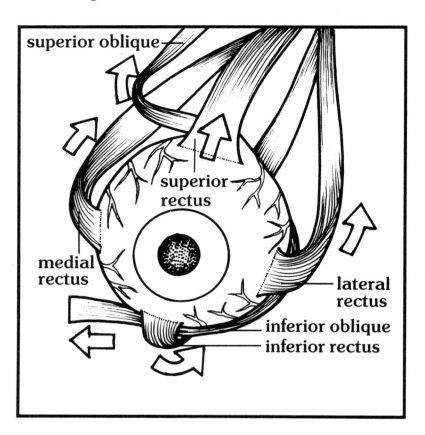

- superior oblique
- superior rectus
- medial rectus
- lateral rectus
- inferior oblique
- inferior rectus

The eye muscles Eye movement is controlled by six muscles inside the eye socket that attach to the sclera, the white outer covering of the eye. Muscles at the top and bottom of the eye pull it up or down. Muscles at either side pull the eye to the left or right. The other two muscles make it possible for the eye to roll in a clockwise or counterclockwise motion.

Eye movements allow the eye to follow moving objects without turning the head. They also make it possible to focus the sharpest light-sensing cells in the middle of the eye on whatever object is being looked at. Generally both eyes *track,* or move, in the same direction at the same time. This is not because the muscles of the right and left eye are attached but because part of the lower brain automatically sends the same message to the muscles of both eyes.

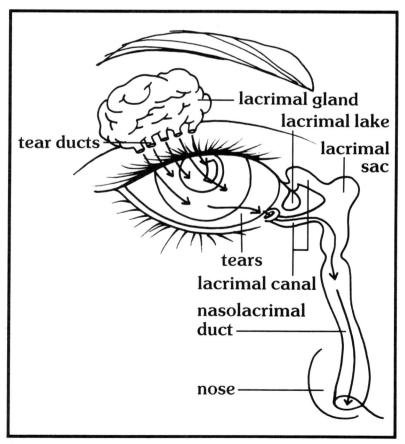

- lacrimal gland
- lacrimal lake
- tear ducts
- lacrimal sac
- tears
- lacrimal canal
- nasolacrimal duct
- nose

Tears The eyes are constantly kept wet with *tears,* a clear fluid mixture of water, salt, mucus, and a chemical that kills bacteria. Tears are made continuously by the *lacrimal glands,* which are located above each eye. Tears come out of several *tear ducts,* are pushed across the eye by blinking, and then flow into the inner corner of the eye. There they pass through a tiny hole into the *lacrimal canal* and collect in the *lacrimal lake.* Finally they flow down the *nasolacrimal ducts,* two tiny tubes that lead to the back of the nose. This is what causes people to blow their noses when they cry or when dirt gets in their eyes.

How the eye focuses

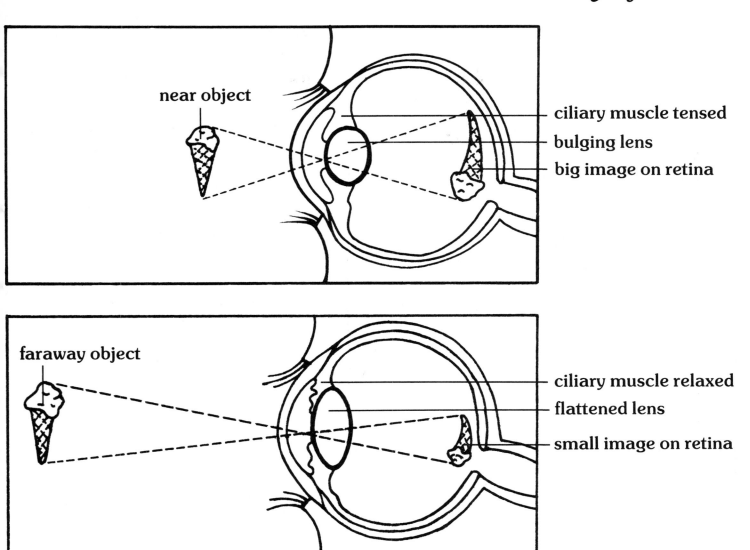

near object — ciliary muscle tensed — bulging lens — big image on retina

faraway object — ciliary muscle relaxed — flattened lens — small image on retina

How the eye focuses   The job of the *lens* is to shrink down an outside scene so that it fits on the *retina* lining the back of the eye. Whenever light rays pass through an outward-bulging curve like the lens, the incoming rays are automatically bent closer together. In order to make the image sharp, the lens must bend the rays just the right amount to make them land exactly on the retina. The closer an object is, the bigger its image looks and the more the light rays coming from it have to be bent. The farther away an image is, the smaller it looks, so the less the light rays have to be bent. The *ciliary muscle* controls the curve of the lens. When an object is near, the brain automatically tightens the ciliary muscle, caus-

ing the lens to bulge more. When an object is far away, the brain relaxes the ciliary muscle, causing the lens to flatten.

The brain has another important role in seeing. As light comes through the lens, the light from the top is bent down and comes out at the bottom of the retina, while the light from the bottom comes out at the top. Thus the whole picture that lands on the retina is not only smaller, it is also upside down. In the brain the image is turned right side up.

The ear

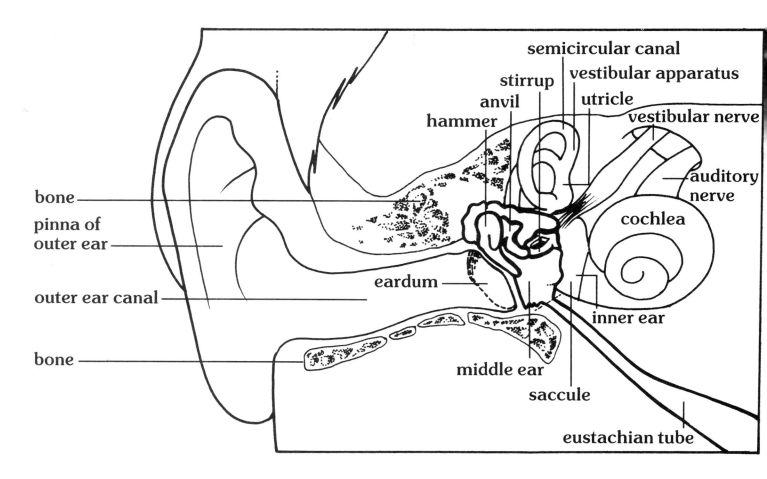

bone

pinna of
outer ear

outer ear canal

bone

hammer

anvil

stirrup

semicircular canal

vestibular apparatus

utricle

vestibular nerve

auditory
nerve

cochlea

eardrum

inner ear

middle ear

saccule

eustachian tube

The ear The *ear* is a special part of the nervous system whose job is to pick up sounds, turn them into nerve impulses, and send them to the brain. Sounds are actually invisible waves that jiggle, or vibrate, the air around them. High sounds vibrate the air quickly, low sounds slowly.

The ear has three major parts. What *we see* is the *outer ear*. It consists of a wrinkly funnel on the outside called the *pinna* and a tube called the *external canal* leading in through the skull. The inner end of this tube is covered with a tightly stretched piece of skin called the *eardrum.*

Beyond the eardrum lies the *middle ear,* a cavelike area whose only opening is to the *eustachian tube,* a tiny tube that leads to the back of the throat. This tube keeps the pressure the same on both sides of the eardrum so that it can vibrate freely when sound waves hit it. The middle ear contains three tiny bones, the *hammer,* the *anvil,*

and the *stirrup.* The last bone touches the *oval window,* the opening to the third part of the ear.

The *inner ear* consists of two hollow spaces in the bones of the skull: the *cochlea,* and the *vestibular apparatus.* The cochlea is the part that helps send sounds to the brain. It is spiral shaped and filled with fluid. Many tiny hairlike nerve endings stick out into this fluid. When a sound vibrates the eardrum, it jiggles the three little bones in the middle ear, which in turn start waves going back and forth in the cochlear fluid. This shakes the nerve hairs and starts a signal that passes along the *auditory nerve* to a special area of the brain. Step by step, the brain figures out which side the sound comes from, whether it is high or low, what the pattern is, and, finally, what it means.

The other part of the inner ear, the vestibular apparatus, helps people keep their balance. It has a central area and three loops called the *semicircular canals*. Each canal tells the brain when the head moves in a different direction. One canal faces sideways, one front-to-back, and one is on its side. Like the cochlea, the canals are filled with fluid and little nerve hairs. When a person's head tilts in any direction, the hairs in one of the canals are rubbed and send off a message to the brain. The center part of the vestibular apparatus contains the *saccule* and the *utricle*. Here nerve hairs are stuck in a Jell-O-like substance that is covered with sandy grains. These nerve cells signal when the head moves suddenly. All messages from the vestibular apparatus pass along the *vestibular nerve* to a special area of the brain. From this information the brain puts muscles to work to keep the body in balance.

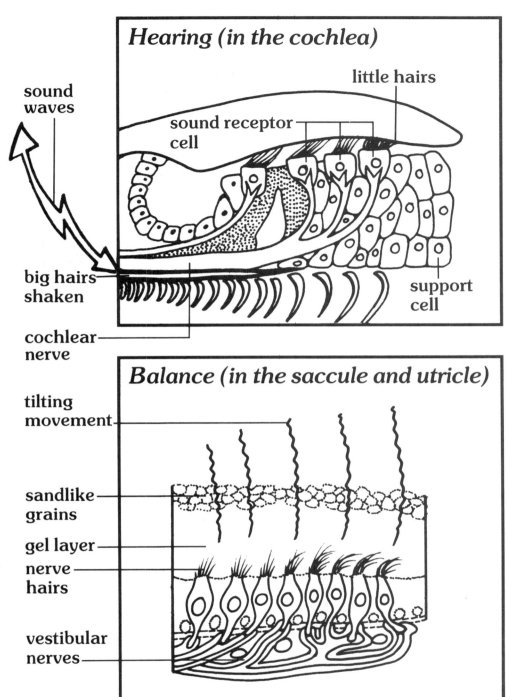

Hearing (in the cochlea)

little hairs

sound waves

sound receptor cell

big hairs shaken

support cell

cochlear nerve

Balance (in the saccule and utricle)

tilting movement

sandlike grains

gel layer

nerve hairs

vestibular nerves

The nose

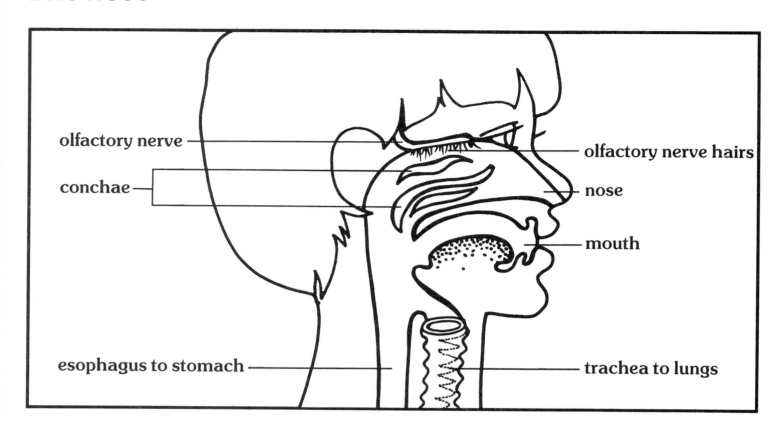

olfactory nerve

conchae

esophagus to stomach

olfactory nerve hairs

nose

mouth

trachea to lungs

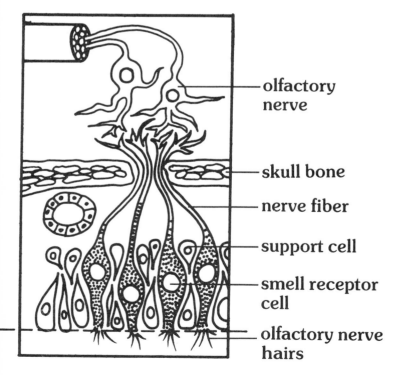

olfactory nerve

skull bone

nerve fiber

support cell

smell receptor cell

olfactory nerve hairs

The nose   The *nose* not only warms, moistens, and filters the air we breathe, it contains the cells that pick up odors or smells. Odors are simply airborne molecules from a substance.

In one square inch at the top of the nose there are 100 million of these special nerve cells. The cells have tiny hairs that stick out into the lining of the nose. When molecules hit these nerve cells, they send messages along the *olfactory nerve* to an area of the brain that identifies odors. When people are breathing ordinarily, they only pick up strong odors because most of the air they inhale goes past the lower *conchae,* the mazelike folds inside the nose. Sniffing helps to identify weaker odors because it brings molecules all the way up to the top of the nose.

The tongue

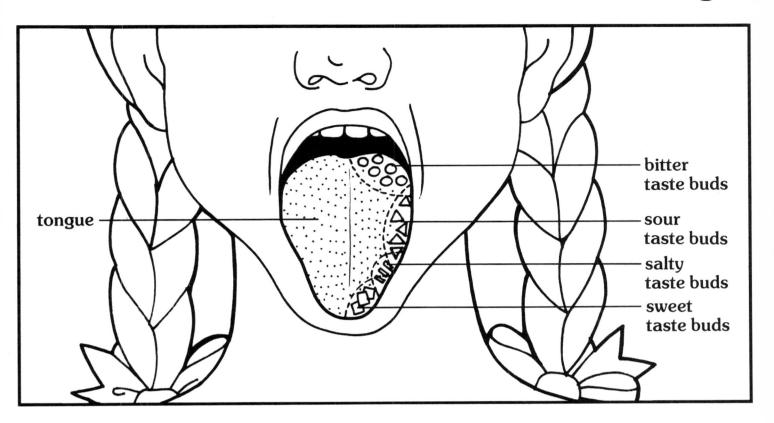

bitter
taste buds

sour
taste buds

salty
taste buds

sweet
taste buds

tongue

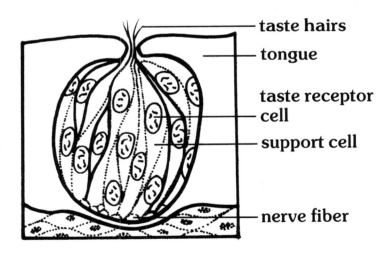

taste hairs

tongue

taste receptor
cell

support cell

nerve fiber

The tongue The *tongue* is not only a muscle that people use in talking and eating, it is a part of the nervous system. The top and sides of the tongue contain 10,000 sensory organs called *taste buds.* Each taste bud is made up of special skin cells with hairlike endings that stick out from the tongue. These endings react to certain chemicals in the mouth and send messages along *nerve fibers* in the bud.

Each taste bud picks up one of four basic kinds of tastes, or flavors: salty, sweet, bitter, or sour. Most taste buds of the same kind are located in the same area of the tongue. Bitter taste buds are in the back of the tongue; sour ones on the sides toward the back; and sweet and salty ones toward the front. The brain learns to recognize different tastes, including ones that are combinations.

The endocrine system

The endocrine system   The *endocrine system* is a group of *glands* throughout the body that control how fast a person grows and makes energy. To do this, the endocrine glands make chemical messengers called *hormones*. Some of these chemicals work throughout the body, some only work in one place. Where they work is determined by which cells have sites that the hormones can lock onto.

The endocrine glands are called the *ductless glands* because they do not store up large amounts of hormones and pour them out all at once. Instead they release the chemicals directly into the bloodstream drop by drop as soon as they are made. This kind of production helps the body function smoothly and steadily. Since the glands do make the hormones constantly, it is easy for them to make a little more or a little less depending on what is needed. A special center in the brain called the *hypothalamus* constantly measures hormone levels and directs these small adjustments.

The *pituitary gland* in the brain is called the *master gland* because its hormones actually control how much the other glands make. The front of the pituitary affects overall growth, plus the thyroid, adrenals, testes, ovaries, and the production of milk after a woman has had a baby. The back of the pituitary makes one hormone that controls how much water the kidneys save and another that causes contractions of the uterus when a baby is born.

The *thyroid gland,* which is located in the neck, makes the hormone that controls overall energy production and children's growth rates. Around the thyroid are four tiny glands called the *parathyroids.* Their hormone controls how much calcium is in the blood to help nerves and muscles work.

The *islets of Langerhans* are special endocrine cells that are scattered throughout the *pancreas,* a long gland that lies under the stomach. The islets make two kinds of hormones that help the body use

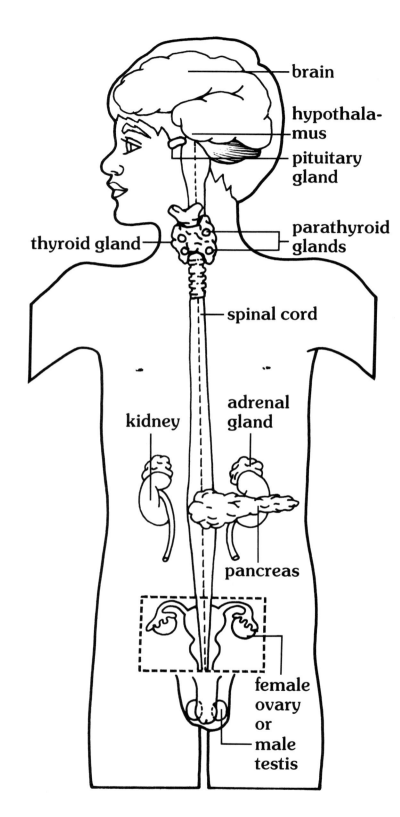

How thoughts affect the endocrine system

sugar for energy production. One hormone, called *insulin,* makes it possible for sugar to pass from the blood into the cells. The other, which is called *glucagon,* makes the liver send out stored sugar when the body needs to do more work.

The *adrenals* are two glands that sit on top of the kidneys. The *cortex,* the outer part of the adrenals, makes two groups of hormones. One group controls the amount of sodium and potassium the kidneys save. The other group determines how much sugar, fat, and protein can be put to work in the body's cells. The inside of each adrenal is called the *medulla.* It makes hormones that control the body's automatic functions such as breathing, heartbeat, and digestion, and determines whether the body is relaxed or on alert.

The *testes* and *ovaries* are the male and female endocrine glands. They produce hormones that control the adolescent growth spurt and cause the changes that make it possible for men and women to create babies.

How thoughts affect the endocrine system

Thoughts in the mind have a great effect on the whole body. Nerve impulses in the brain directly affect the *hypothalamus* and the part of the nervous system that controls automatic functions like breathing. In particular, feelings of excitement or alarm send signals along the *sympathetic nerves* to the adrenals. These feelings cause the *adrenal medullae* to produce hormones that result in a burst of energy. People find that their heart beats faster, they begin to sweat, and they feel flutters in their stomach. Calm, peaceful thoughts cause the opposite things to happen. Feelings such as these send signals along the *parasympathetic nerves,* causing the heart to slow down, the digestive system to work harder, and the other muscles to relax.

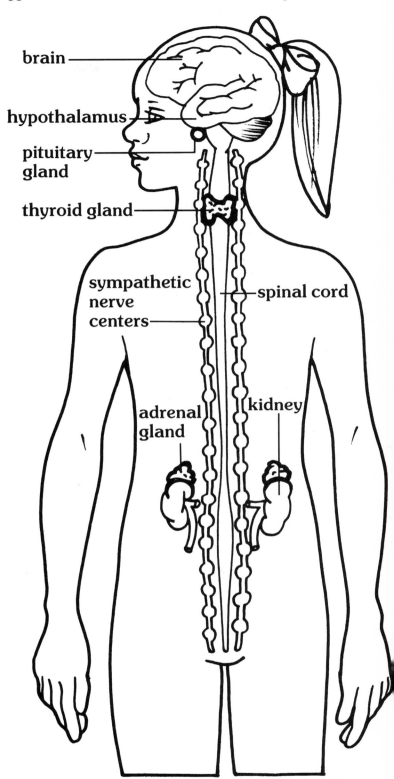

brain

hypothalamus

pituitary gland

thyroid gland

sympathetic nerve centers

spinal cord

adrenal gland

kidney

The female reproductive system

The female reproductive system
The *female reproductive system* makes it possible for a woman to become a mother. Eggs are made in the *ovaries,* two tiny organs in a girl's abdomen. The eggs are all formed before girls are born, but they don't begin to mature for about ten years. Then once a month an egg pops out of an ovary and is guided into the end of the *fallopian tube* by a fingerlike *fimbria.* This process is called *ovulation.*

It is in the fallopian tube that a sperm may join the egg and begin the growth of a baby. This process is called *fertilization.* From the tube, the egg is squeezed into the *uterus,* a pear-shaped organ that can shelter a fertilized egg as it grows into a baby. To prepare for this possibility, the uterus develops a special lining every month. If the egg has not been fertilized, several weeks later both the egg and the lining are washed out through the *cervix,* a narrow opening at the bottom of the uterus. The cervix opens into the *vagina,* a short tube that leads to the outside of the body. The process of releasing the egg and lining is called *menstruation.* It produces a red fluid—because of the blood that was in the lining—for five or six days. Once menstruation is over, egg production begins again. The entire cycle is controlled by two hormones from the brain's pituitary gland, together with two hormones from the ovaries.

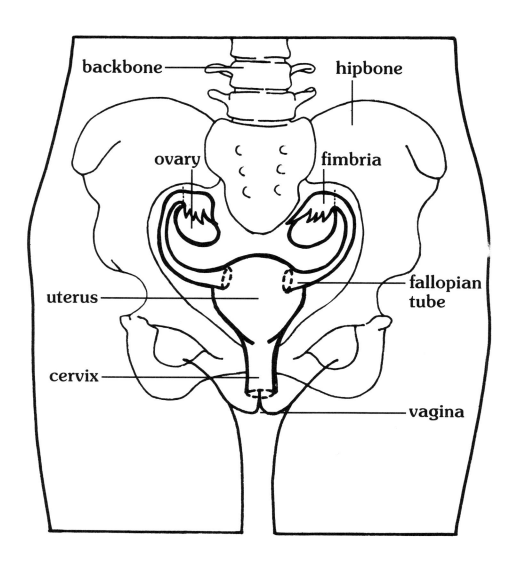

The male reproductive system
The *male reproductive system* makes it possible for a man to become a father. *Sperm,* the male counterpart of female eggs, are made in the *seminiferous tubules* inside two glands called the *testes.* The testes lie in the *scrotum,* a special sac that hangs between boys' legs. Being outside the body keeps sperm several degrees cooler, which is important to their survival. From the seminiferous tubule, the sperm move on into the *epididymus.* In this coiled tube they take several days to finish growing up. Then the sperm travel through a straight tube known as the *vas deferens.* The vas deferens opens into a wide area called the *ampulla.* Here the sperm are temporarily stored. Next to each ampulla is a *seminal vesicle,* which makes food to keep the sperm alive. Below the seminal vesicles is the *prostrate gland,* where a milky fluid is made. The ampullae, seminal vesicles, and prostate all open into the *urethra.* This tube runs from the tip of the *bladder* to the outside of the *penis.* In the urethra, the fluids from the seminal vesicles and prostate combine with sperm. The mixture is called *semen.* Sperm does not start to be formed until boys are 10 to 14 years old. Its production is controlled by two hormones from the brain's pituitary and one from the testes.

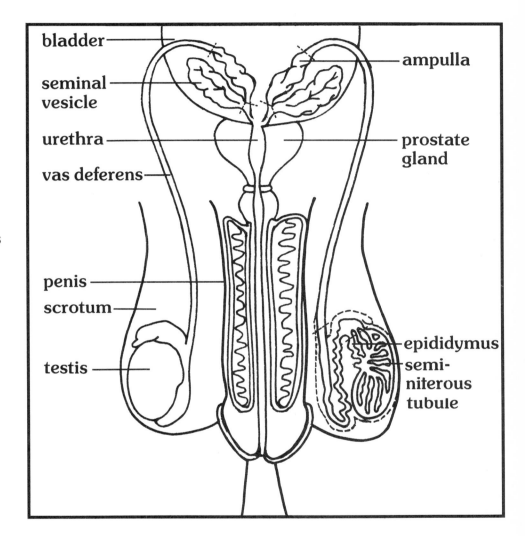

bladder

seminal vesicle

urethra

vas deferens

penis

scrotum

testis

ampulla

prostate gland

epididymus

semi-niterous tubule

Puberty

Puberty Puberty is the time when both girls' and boys' bodies and reproductive organs begin to mature. The reproductive organs are formed before birth, but they don't begin to work or grow in size for about ten years. The exact age at which changes begin to take place inside and outside the body varies greatly from one child to another. Whether changes begin early or late, boys and girls follow a general sequence.

Changes first start deep within the brain when the hypothalamus signals the pituitary gland. It in turn causes girls' *ova-*ries to make *estrogen,* and boys' *testes* to make *testosterone.* These are the hormones that cause an overall spurt in body growth. Over the next few years estrogen and testosterone cause the reproductive organs to grow and start making adult eggs and sperm. These hormones also lead to great changes in girls' and boys' emotional feelings and interests. And finally, the hormones cause dramatic changes in girls' and boys' outside appearance.

In girls the external changes begin with enlargement of the breasts and nipples. During the general growth spurt that follows, girls' hips grow wider and heavier, and they grow darker, thicker hair under their arms and around their vagina. Meanwhile, other changes take place inside that cause an egg to pop out of an ovary once a month and pass into the uterus. If this egg is not joined by a sperm, both the egg

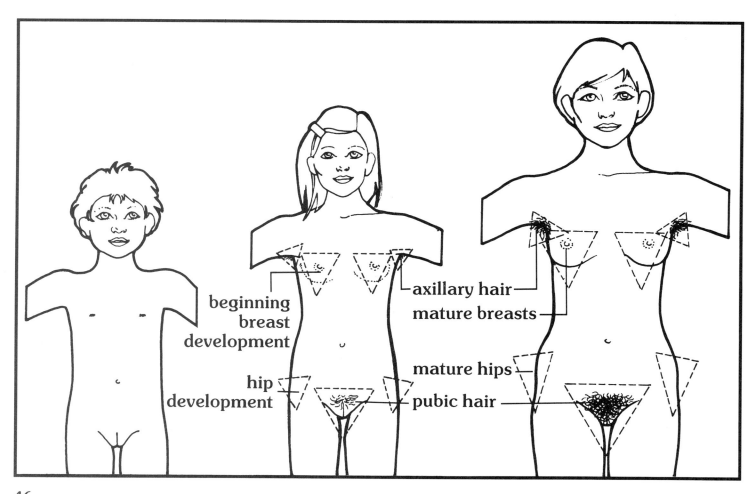

beginning breast development

hip development

axillary hair
mature breasts

mature hips
pubic hair

and a special lining of the uterus are cast off over a period of five or six days. This process, called *menstruation,* generally begins at around 12 or 13 but can start several years earlier or later.

In boys, the changes of puberty begin outside with growth of the testes and scrotum and inside with the making of sperm. Somewhat later the penis begins to increase in size. These changes are followed by an over-all growth spurt sometime between the ages of 11 and 16. During this spurt, boys not only grow taller, their muscles grow larger, especially in the shoulder area, and their bones become thicker and heavier. Boys' voice boxes also grow larger, which causes occasional cracking and then deepening of their voices. Finally, boys begin to grow thicker, darker hair around their penis, armpits, chest, and face.

All of the changes of puberty happen gradually over a number of years. Changes generally begin a little earlier in girls and take a little longer in boys. The earlier they start, the sooner they tend to be completed in both boys and girls.

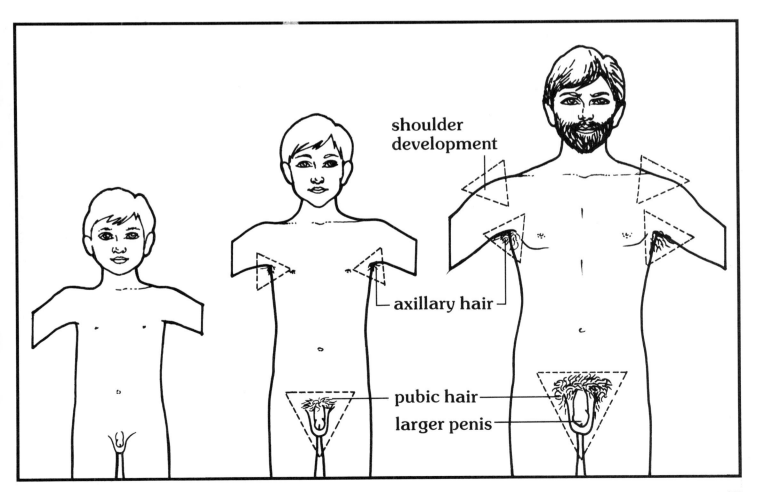

shoulder development

axillary hair

pubic hair
larger penis

Fertilization of an egg

Fertilization of an egg A baby is formed by the joining of two special cells, an egg from the mother and a sperm from the father. Each contains only half the information stored in a regular cell. When they join, they become a complete cell unlike any other. A baby isn't a copy of its mother or father but a mixture of both.

Chemicals in the sperm dissolve the wall of the egg, and the sperm enters and joins its 23 *chromosomes* with the 23 from the egg. This process, called *fertilization*, usually takes place in the mother's fallopian tube, where the sperm swims from the vagina.

For more than a day the fertilized egg readies itself for changes. Then it begins to divide and make new cells every 15 hours. In the first three days the egg moves from the fallopian tube into the uterus. By this point the egg has formed a ball of cells. On the next day, the ball has formed a hollow center.

At first the fertilized egg floats freely in the uterus, but by the seventh day it begins to burrow into the thickened wall of the uterus. For quite a while the egg is fed by a fluid called *uterine milk,* which is made by tiny glands in the lining of the uterus.

Meanwhile cells in the egg have started to become different from each other. One group of cells starts to form the baby, or *embryo,* itself. By the 14th day it has already developed a beginning head and beginning heart. Another group of cells starts to form the *placenta,* a special organ that attaches to the uterine wall. It is also attached to the baby's belly button by the *umbilical cord.* The placenta eventually becomes the means by which the mother's body feeds the baby for the last six months until its birth.

48

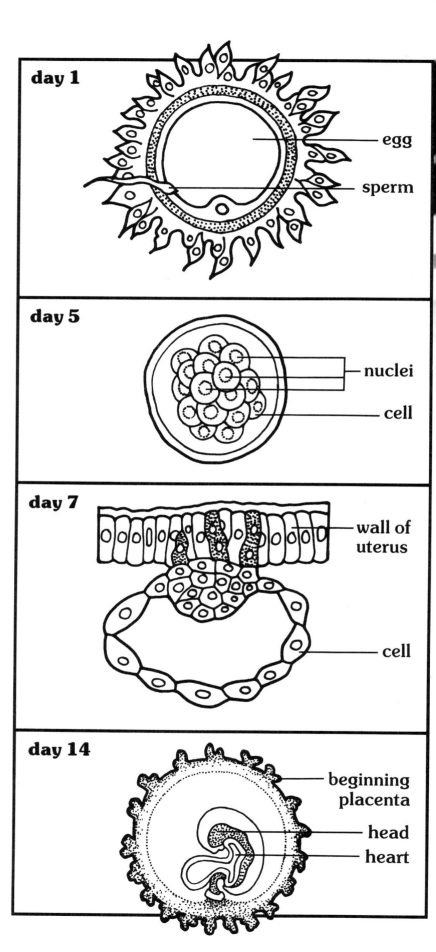

Growth of a baby All the organs and parts of the growing baby, or *embryo,* are basically formed by the end of eight weeks. The baby even looks human, but it is only one inch long and weighs almost nothing.

By this time the *placenta* is almost fully formed. It attaches to the baby's belly button by the *umbilical cord.* Through this cord the baby's blood circulates between its body and the placenta. In the placenta the baby's blood is separated from the mother's by only the thinnest wall. Molecules of food and oxygen cross into the baby's blood and molecules of carbon dioxide and other wastes are carried off by the mother's blood. So the placenta both breathes for and feeds the growing baby.

During the next several months the baby's organs become more complete and it floats freely in the *amniotic fluid* filling the uterus. By the sixth month the baby is 14 inches long and weighs about two and a half pounds.

In the last months the baby grows rapidly in length and weight, stretching the mother's uterus and abdomen. In the weeks before birth, the baby becomes so large that it lies curled up with its arms and legs folded against its chest. Generally its head is now down, and this is the position in which most babies are born.

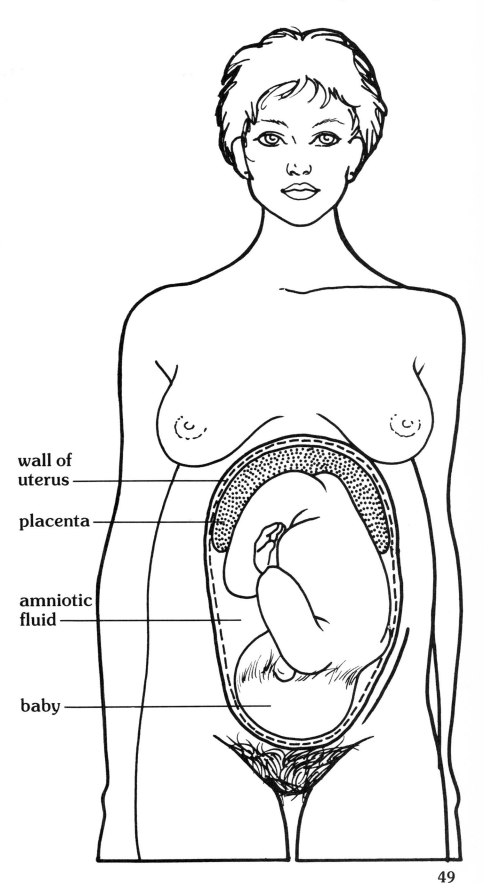

wall of uterus

placenta

amniotic fluid

baby

Blood clotting

when a cut occurs

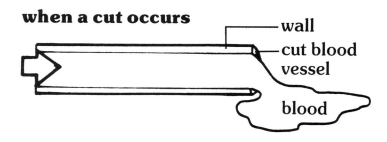

wall
cut blood vessel
blood

within fifteen seconds

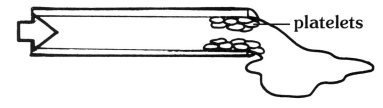

platelets

within a minute

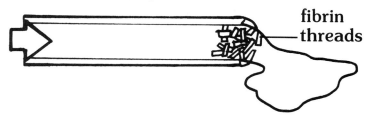

fibrin threads

within six minutes

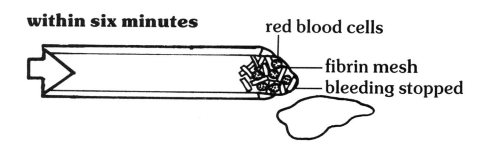

red blood cells
fibrin mesh
bleeding stopped

within twenty minutes after clotting

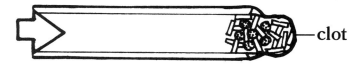

clot

Blood clotting The body is filled with millions of tiny blood vessels. When a person gets a cut, the walls of some of these vessels are broken. Muscles in the blood vessels' walls immediately tighten and slow the bleeding. Tiny *collagen fibers* stick out from the ends of the cut blood vessels. When *platelets,* which are tiny white blood cells, bump into the collagen fibers, something remarkable happens. Within seconds the platelets swell, become sticky, and start to clump together, blocking the holes in the blood vessels.

In bigger cuts, the blood itself has to clot. Clotting requires *fibrinogen,* a protein in the watery part of the blood. A special chemical at the site of the cut causes the fibrinogen to join into long threads, which form a mesh across the break. Blood cells and more platelets are caught in the net and together they form a *clot.* About 20 minutes after a clot forms it actually shrinks a little, closing the hole even more tightly.

Pressure from the outside helps to slow or stop bleeding and keeps a clot from washing out, but it doesn't speed the clotting time. That varies from one person to another and depends on how fast the chemicals in the blood work. In small cuts, clotting generally begins in about 15 seconds and stops the bleeding in 3 to 6 minutes.

Skin healing   The body begins to heal a cut immediately. Within minutes the blood clots at the break in the blood vessel. Broken cells in the area release a chemical called *histamine*. It widens blood vessels to bring more blood into the area and lets more *plasma*, the clear watery part of the blood, leak out into the spaces between the cells. Plasma contains the protein *fibrinogen*, which forms into threads that clump, or clot. Clotting plasma causes the swelling around a cut and helps keep germs from spreading.

At the same time, chemicals released by the injured cells alert *white blood cells* and bring them to the area in large numbers. These cells immediately begin to *phagocytize*, or eat, damaged cells and germs in the area. Cells of another kind, the *fibroblasts*, also move into the cut area. These cells make *collagen fibers*, tough threads that hold together the sides of a cut.

Meanwhile, cells in the *epidermis*, the top layer of skin, start forming new cells at 20 times their usual rate. These new cells rapidly roll over one another and grow under the scab right down into the cut. When they meet at the bottom, they stop forming new cells.

In as little as six hours the broken blood vessels begin to grow many new endings. These endings eventually grow directly into the clot and join new endings growing from the other side.

Healing can take anywhere from several days to several weeks depending on what a cut is like. Because a cut heals from side to side, it really does not take any longer to heal if it is one inch or three inches long. What is important is how deep the cut is and where it is. Doctors put in stitches if cuts are long and deep or are in areas of movement. Stitches do not speed healing, but they keep the cut from reopening, and they leave less of a scar.

within minutes after a cut

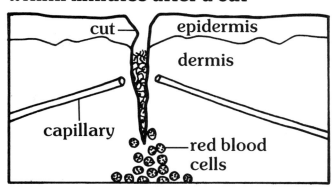

six to forty-eight hours after a cut

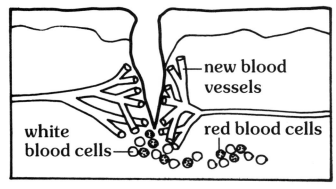

two to fourteen days after a cut

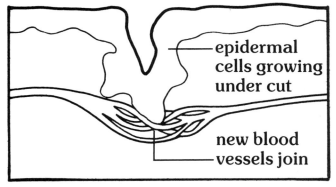

two weeks after a cut

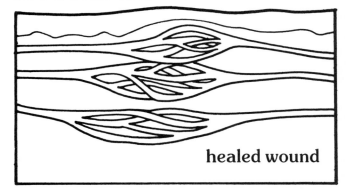

Bone healing

broken bone

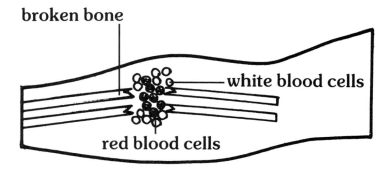

white blood cells

red blood cells

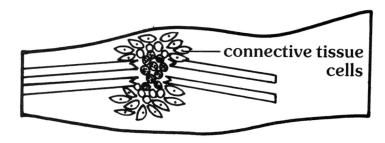

connective tissue cells

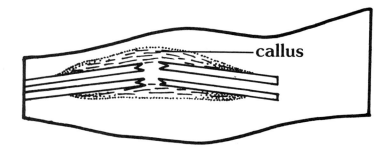

callus

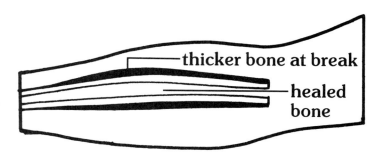

thicker bone at break

healed bone

Bone healing When a bone breaks, many blood vessels break inside even if the skin is not broken. Until clotting takes place, blood leaks out into the spaces between the cells. This is what causes bruises and discoloration. Special proteins in *plasma,* the watery part of the blood, form clots between the cells and cause swelling around the break. As with any cut, the broken blood vessels gradually form a new network. And *white blood cells* come into the area and begin to eat up bacteria, dead cells, and clotted plasma.

Within a day or so, *connective tissue cells* start dividing rapidly and filling the area around the broken ends of the bone. These cells later change into one of three kinds of cells that do special jobs. Some turn into *osteoblasts* and make new bone cells; some turn into *chondroblasts* and make new cartilage cells; and some turn into *fibroblasts* and make new connective tissue fibers. In the center of the break, osteoblasts make a rough bone bridge consisting of collagen fibers with calcium crystals stuck to them. Around this bridge, chondroblasts make a layer of rubbery cartilage. This whole mass is called a *callus.* It acts like a splint, or brace, and keeps the broken ends of the bone from moving. Over a period of weeks, hard bone is laid down where it is needed, and extra cells in the callus are dissolved.

Doctors put a cast on a broken bone because it helps to keep the ends in line, not because it makes the bone heal faster. Even after the cast is removed, the broken bone continues to change. Bone cells are added or removed depending on the forces on the bone. In a young person the callus around the break disappears completely by six months, and it can become hard to tell the bone has ever been broken.

How antibodies destroy bacteria

How antibodies destroy bacteria *Antibodies* are substances made by white blood cells to fight germs or poisons from outside the body. Each kind of antibody is shaped to lock onto the surface of just one kind of *bacteria,* or dangerous substance. In *plasma,* the watery part of the blood, there are chemicals called *complement enzymes,* which work with antibodies. When these enzymes come in contact with antibodies attached to bacteria, they cover the bacteria and make them stick together in clumps. The complement also begins to dissolve hooks on the outside of the bacteria and even the *cell membrane* of the bacteria. Then cell fluid rushes in, pressure builds up, and the bacteria explode. Finally, other white blood cells come in and eat up the pieces.

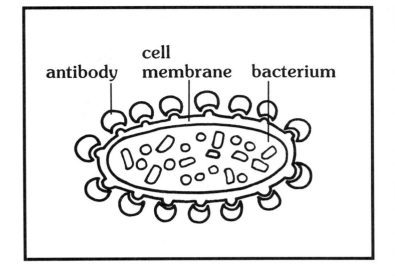

antibody   cell membrane   bacterium

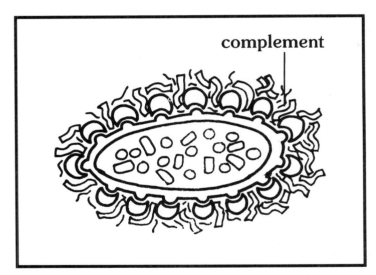

complement

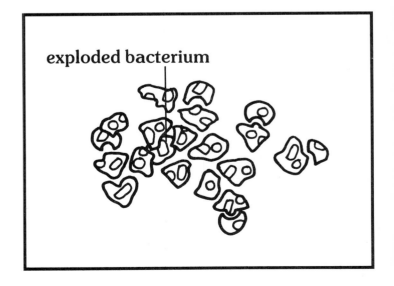

exploded bacterium

How stress affects the body

How stress affects the body
People's thoughts affect how their bodies work and feel. The brain is connected to all parts of the body by nerves and by chemical messengers called *hormones*. Whenever people are scared or worried, a part of their brain called the *hypothalamus* sends many messages out through the *sympathetic nerves*. These messages cause heartbeat, breathing, blood pressure, and sweating to speed up and digestion and cell repair to slow down. All these body reactions are good if you need to run away from a poisonous snake, but they aren't good if they happen all the time. They wear down the body and give it less energy for healing.

Whether a scary thought is real doesn't matter. A rope that looks like a snake or a dream about a snake can be just as frightening as a real snake. You know this is true if you think about how you react to a frightening movie: Your body becomes tense, your breath sticks in your throat, and your stomach gets knots in it. If kids learn to recognize and deal with stressful thoughts and fears, they can become happier and make their bodies healthier.

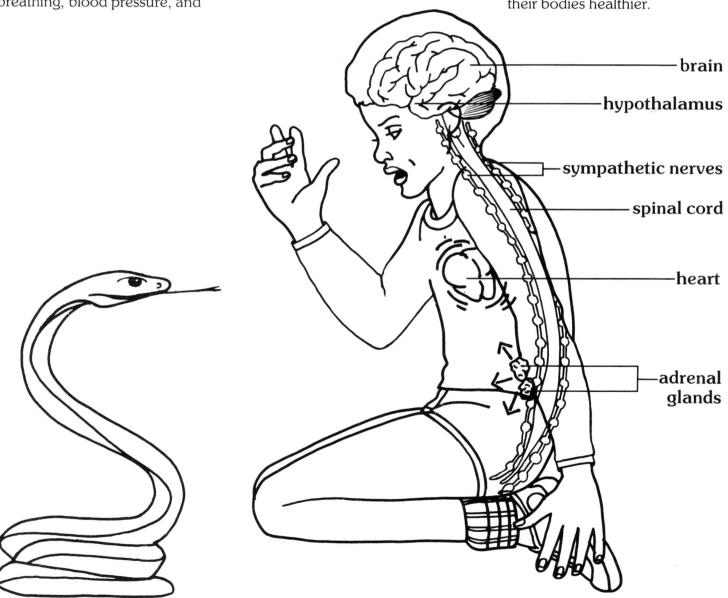

brain

hypothalamus

sympathetic nerves

spinal cord

heart

adrenal glands

How relaxation affects the body

How relaxation affects the body
When people have peaceful or happy thoughts, it affects how their body feels and works. A part of the brain called the *hypothalamus* sends fewer messages out through the sympathetic nerves and more through the *parasympathetic nerves.* They cause the body to relax and rest. Heartbeat and breathing slow down. The body's energy is directed to breaking down food, making cells, and fighting germs.

Just as the body cannot tell the difference between scary thoughts that are real or imagined, it does not matter if "good" things are really happening to a person as long as the person feels happy. For example, one child might be unhappy because the vacation is half over. Another child might be happy because there is still half the vacation to go. Both kids have the same amount of time left, but one is happy and the other is not. With practice anybody can learn to concentrate on the good things in life and the things they enjoy.

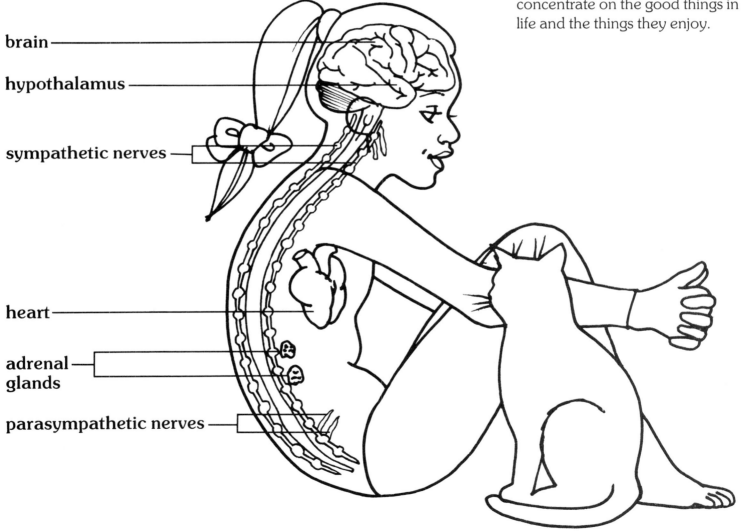

brain

hypothalamus

sympathetic nerves

heart

adrenal glands

parasympathetic nerves

How to relax

How to relax Kids can learn how to relax and make their bodies healthier just by giving their muscles instructions to relax. The muscles actually get their instructions from the mind all the time, but people usually are not aware of it. Your arm does not wave by itself, you have to think, ''I'm going to wave to my friends.''

The first step in learning how to relax is learning what *tension* feels like. Tension is the opposite of relaxation. Muscles tense when they are working and relax when they are at rest. Often people do not realize that their muscles remain a little tense even when they are not working. This tension wastes energy and can make people sick.

Here is an easy way to feel the difference between tension and relaxation. Rest your arm on a table. Then bend your hand up slightly at the wrist. Feel the tension in your forearm. It feels hot and tight. Now let your hand drop. That's relaxation.

To practice relaxation, sit or lie in a comfortable position. Breathe in and out slowly and evenly. Say to yourself, ''My feet are relaxing.'' Rest and let them relax. One by one, tell your legs, hips, stomach, back, and chest to relax in the same way. Now tell your arms, neck, jaws, and eyes to relax. Then rest and enjoy the easy, floppy feeling.

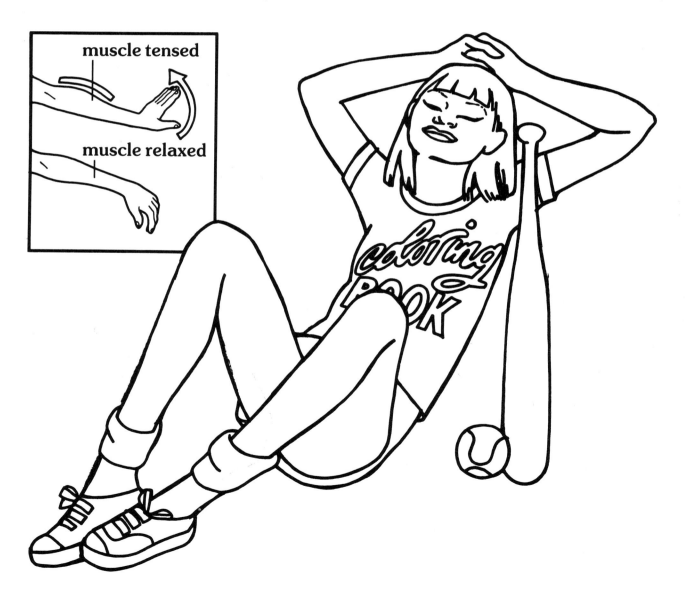

muscle tensed

muscle relaxed

How to use mind pictures

How to use mind pictures
Thoughts that people hold in their minds have real effects on their bodies. Doctors have found that if you picture an ice cube in your hand, the temperature of that hand will actually drop. When you picture a scene vividly, your mind can't tell if you're really seeing it or simply imagining it.

Mind pictures are just day-dreaming on purpose. And these daydreams can be very useful. They can help you get rid of scary thoughts; they can help you do better at school or in sports; and they can help you to be more creative. They can even help you to cure yourself when you are sick or have a stomach-ache or headache because you are upset.

Many school coaches have kids picture doing different sports movements to help them to improve their performance. Mind pictures are just another way of practicing. Even though you may not feel it, the same nerve cells in the brain and muscles that are excited by roller-skating are excited by imagining roller-skating.

To try using mind pictures, sit in a quiet place in a comfortable position. Close your eyes. Breathe in and out slowly. Concentrate on relaxing for a minute. Then try and picture what you want to be better at. Imagine the kind of clothes you usually wear and the place where you practice. See the people you work with. Picture the movements you make, the equipment you use. Go over and over your pictures until you get them exactly right in your mind. The clearer your mind pictures and the more often you practice them, the better you will become.

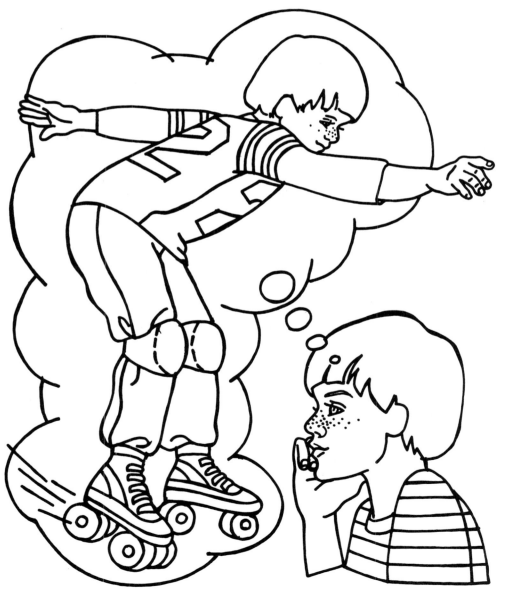

Healthy eating

Healthy eating Your whole body is made of molecules from the food you eat. You use food to make energy, to grow, and to replace old cells. Your body needs five basic kinds of foods to do different jobs. If your body gets too much or too little of them, growth can be affected or your body can become sick.

The body gets its energy from *carbohydrates* and *fats*. Fats are in butter, oil, meat, and cheese. Carbohydrates are found in bread, cereal, corn, potatoes, spaghetti, and desserts. Carbohydrates are made of *sugars* and *starches*.

The building blocks for the body come from *proteins, vitamins,* and *minerals*. All the cells in the body, as well as hormones, antibodies, and digestive enzymes, are made of protein. Protein is found in milk, cheese, nuts, eggs, meat, fish, chicken, corn, beans, rice, and bread. Vitamins and minerals are chemicals the body needs to do special jobs. They help regulate body fluids, aid digestion, make nerves and muscles work, help red blood cells carry oxygen, and help make certain hormones and enzymes. Vitamins and minerals are found in fruits, vegetables, and meat.

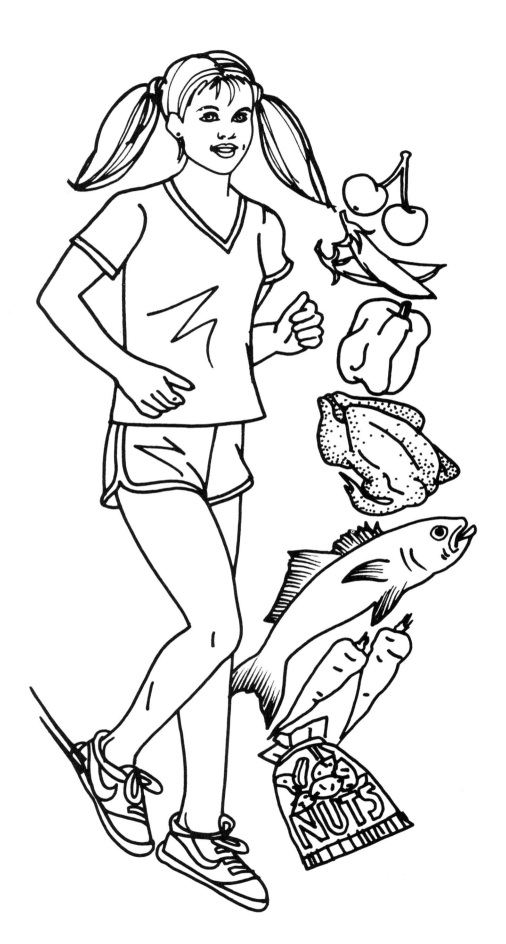

Unhealthy eating   A number of foods don't have many proteins, minerals, or vitamins. Food experts call these *empty foods.* Some empty foods like candy bars and sodas contain mostly sugar. Sugar gives you quick energy, but it does not make you grow. Other empty foods, like white bread, have lost their vitamins and minerals because their ingredients have been heated and ground up so much. These foods are called highly *processed.* Processed foods contain very little *roughage,* or *cellulose,* tough indigestible fibers that help the digestive system work well. Often processed foods are also loaded with chemical colorings, flavorings, and preservatives. Some of these chemicals are bad for the body.

Unfortunately, your stomach fills up just as much on empty foods as it does on foods that are rich in the basic nutrients. Filling up on junk foods can actually make you sick, both now and when you are older. Too much fat causes people to become overweight and increases their chances of getting heart disease later on. Too much salt can lead to high blood pressure in some people. And too much sugar makes people fat and gives them cavities.

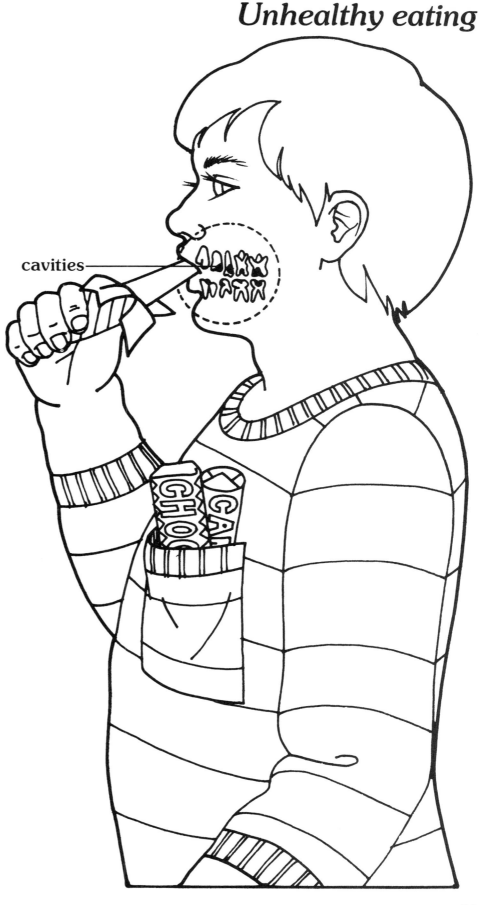

cavities

Body pollution

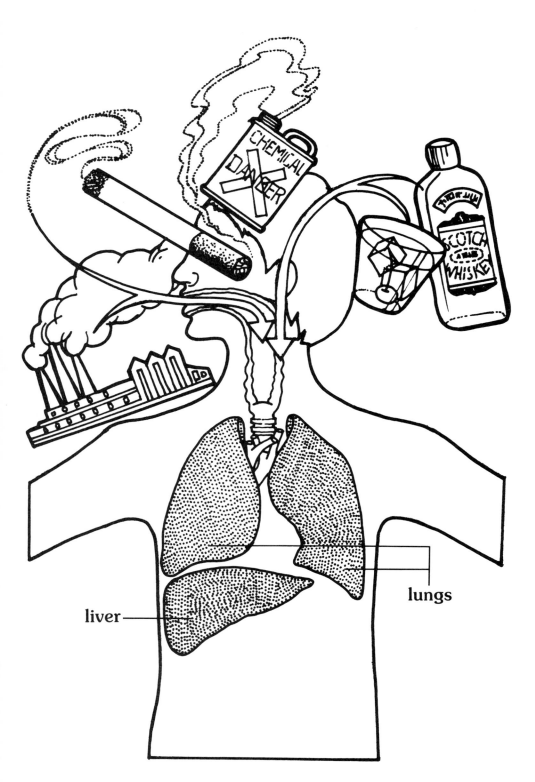

liver

lungs

Body pollution Many chemicals in the environment are now known to be harmful to our bodies. Some of these chemicals are found in foods we eat, beverages we drink, air we breathe, and products we buy.

Many things that aren't good for the body are substancess that people choose to use for "fun." Some may not be too harmful if people do not use them much, but they become unhealthy if used a lot.

Smoking is one of the worst health hazards. Chemicals in cigarette smoke irritate the lining of the lungs and clog the air sacs. Smokers get less oxygen when they breathe, so their hearts and lungs have to work harder all the time. Heavy smokers have much higher rates of lung cancer and heart disease.

Beer, wine, and hard liquor all contain *alcohol*. Getting drunk damages the digestive system and causes problems with coordination that lead to a large number of car accidents. Chronic heavy drinking injures the liver and can even kill people.

Many chemicals used in medicine, industry, and the home are being found to be dangerous. Some chemicals cause illness immediately, but many take years to make people sick.

How aerobic exercise affects the body When kids run, bike, or swim, they are using their big muscles over and over in a regular pattern. To do this kind of work, muscle fibers need oxygen and glucose, a special kind of sugar. As a result of working, muscles produce carbon dioxide and other waste products. Muscles become "tired" when the blood cannot bring in new supplies and take away wastes fast enough. The amount of work muscles can do depends on how hard the heart can pump, how much air the lungs can take in, and how many blood vessels muscles have developed.

Kids who get little exercise tire very quickly. The more kids exercise, the stronger and bigger their hearts, lungs, blood vessels, and muscles become. Steady, hard exercise over a period of 15 or 20 minutes is called *aerobic exercise*. When this kind of exercise is done three or four days a week over a period of months, it will actually produce lifelong changes. In fact, adults who have done aerobic training as kids will always be able to do more work than adults who never trained as kids. The biggest changes can only take place while kids are still growing.

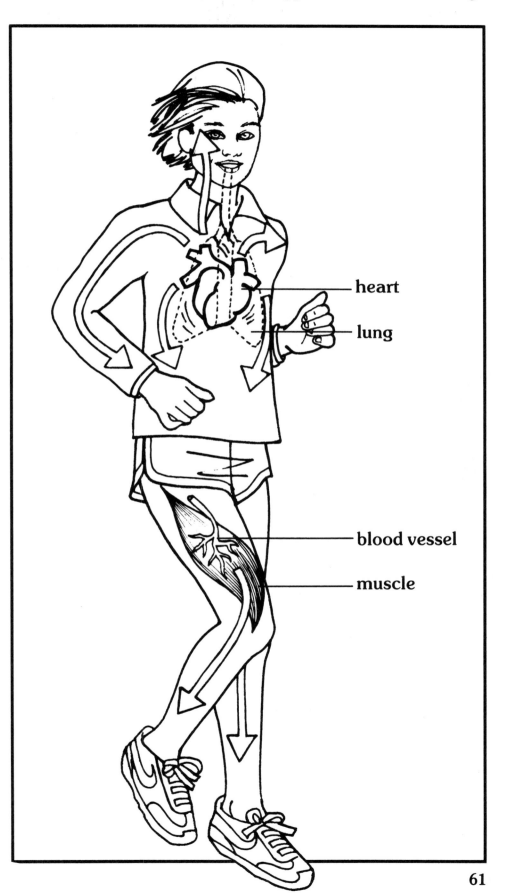

heart

lung

blood vessel

muscle

Feeling good

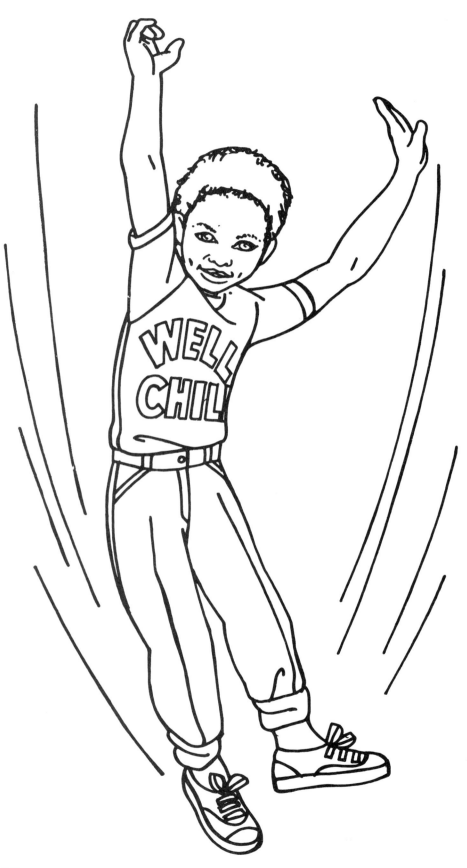

Feeling good   Children's health is affected by their whole world. When children eat food that helps to make energy and new cells, they grow and stay healthy. When they breathe clean air and drink pure water, they keep healthy. When children get lots of exercise, their hearts, lungs, muscles, and bones grow big and strong. When children are happy and relaxed, their brains send messages to their bodies to make repairs and stop infections. The environment is filled with bacteria and viruses, but generally people are healthy. They only get sick when their white blood cells cannot keep up with the germs.

Children can actually do a lot to keep themselves healthy. They can learn what foods are good for their bodies and make a habit of eating them. They can learn how important exercise is and make it a part of their lives. They can learn to relax and do things that make them feel proud and happy. The more children concentrate on thinking and feeling healthy, the healthier they are likely to be.